Surgical Eponyms

For General Surgery FRCS, MRCS, European and American Board Exams

Hutan Ashrafian

INSTITUTE OF CIVILISATION PRESS

London, UK

ISBN: 1999798236
ISBN-13: 978-1-9997982-3-9

DEDICATION

To my wonderful wife Leanne and delightful son Persie

Hutan Ashrafian

Disclaimer

The topics addressed in this book cover an ever-changing field. The author has made every effort to provide information that is accurate and complete as of the date of publication. However, in view of the rapid changes occurring in medical science, as well as the possibility of human error, this book may contain technical inaccuracies, typographical or other errors.

This book is not intended to be a substitute for the medical advice of a licensed doctor/ surgeon/ physician. The reader should consult with their doctor in any matters relating to his/her health or with an appropriately trained and licensed colleague with regard to healthcare practitioners for any matters relating to patient care.

The information contained herein is provided "as is" is merely information and without warranty of any kind. The author and publisher disclaim responsibility for any errors or omissions or for results obtained from the use of information contained herein.

Table of Contents

PREFACE

Eponyms in surgery and medicine remain a common facet of modern healthcare practice. They represent the naming of a disease, procedure, device or treatment guideline according to a specific named person, group of people, or society. There is however a large paradox in modern healthcare; whilst the advent of evidence-based medicine has been developed on a wave of increased objectivism and 'scientificism' where conditions need accurate descriptions according to scientific principles, the vast majority of clinicians still adhere to the eponyms that have been taught to them throughout their student and clinical careers. In fact, eponyms continue to promulgated in each generation even though the medical and academic establishment suggest that eponyms should be for ever expelled.

This adoration for eponyms may occur for several reasons. These include:

(1) It is easier to communicate and verbalise a single name when describing a complex condition or procedure rather having to didactically describe a disease that has 'so and so' genetics and 'such and such' symptoms.
(2) Following on, it is easier to remember a single name as an aide-memoire that represents a complex underlying principle of a disease or procure rather than memorising multiple facts in one group
(3) In some cases the eponym can offer a deeper association, context or history to the concept with which it is associated. For example the Billroth operation reflects on the era where Northern European surgeons were pioneering abdominal surgery. Alternatively the Aztec Thoarcotomy (or Ashrafian Thoracotomy) offers insight into use of thoracotomy techniques by the Aztecs approximately 5 centuries ago.

(4) There remains the element of vanity by the person who names something after himself or herself, or alternatively respect for someone who names something after another individual or colleague who innovated with a new procedure or a new description of a disease

(5) At a philosophical level, the brilliant 20th century philosopher Ludwig Wittgenstein (1889-1951) suggested in his *Philosophical Investigations* that the structure of language reflects how we think. Consequently the use of a word (and therefore an eponym) is akin to a tool that reflects what you can do with it. As a result, an eponym in a medical description can offer a strong message for how we communicate complex meanings.

(6) Sometimes therefore, naming a disease can give it a stronger strength of societal and political recognition whereas a 'purely scientific' description may fail to express the impact or societal weight of a disorder

(7) Trying to eradicate eponyms from the language of medicine and surgery may be as hard as removing all words with either a French or Latin origin from the English language. These two have been considered to each offer approximately 29% of words in modern English so that eliminating either of them may not be practicable.

Interestingly, the concept of eponyms has only really been in practice since the 18th century following the period of the enlightenment when the classification of all things had become favoured and adopted throughout the scientific establishment. This was prominently exemplified by Carl Linnaeus' system of binomial nomenclature for classifying all organisms. Such a culture became so profound and broadly accepted that it almost became assumed that these classification systems had been present throughout history, and therefore sometimes (though rarely) eponyms where ascribed to ancient physicians thousands of years after the disease or pathology had been described. An example of this is *Celsus' criteria for inflammation* (rubor, tumor, calor and dolor) that were named after Aulus Cornelius Celsus (c.25 BC–c.50 AD).

Invariably some signs, diseases, conditions and techniques were eponymously named after more than one person or authority; in these cases I have specified what they are 'also known as' by listing them sequentially with 'AKA' before each term so that the reader can appreciate the multitude of eponymous terms used in each case.

The study of eponyms became particularly relevant to me during study for surgical exams where an informal poll led to the finding that approximately 20-25% of all post-graduate surgical multiple-choice questions mentioned an eponymous condition. I have therefore complied this book for all those in a similar situation or those who are simply interested and exposed to the persistence of eponyms in general surgery.

Hutan Ashrafian
Primrose Hill
London 2018

1. ANATOMY

Allan Burn's ligament AKA Burn's ligament – (superior falciform margin of the fascia lata opening) where the greater saphenous vein penetrates/ is surrounded by the cribriform fascia before entering the femoral vein in the femoral triangle

Anatomical snuff box AKA snuffbox AKA Tabatière – formed by the scaphoid and trapezium bones at its floor. Contains the origin of the cephalic vein, has within it the radial artery and its skin is supplied by the dorsal cutaneous branch of the radial nerve

Ampulla of Vater AKA Hepatopancreatic ampulla – amalgamation between the common bile duct and the pancreatic duct at the major duodenal papilla

Bell (Long Thoracic Nerve of) AKA External respiratory nerve of Bell AKA Posterior thoracic nerve) – nerve to serratus anterior muscle

Belsey's Fat – Fat pad at the anterior oesophago-gastric junction

Buck's fascia AKA Gallaudet's fascia AKA – deep fascia of the penis

Bühler's anastamotic artery AKA arc of Bühler – Vertical arterial shunt between the coeliac axis and the superior mesenteric artery (SMA)

Camper's Fascia – Superficial tissue of the anterior abdominal wall (superficial to Scarpa's fascia)

Chief cells – (1) stomach, (2) parathyroid, (3) type 1 chief cells of the carotid body

Colles' fascia – membranous layer of the superficial fascia of the perineum (stratum membranosum) that is a continuation Scarpa's fascia from the abdomen

Cooper's ligaments (of the breast) AKA suspensory ligaments of Cooper AKA fibrocollagenous septa – structural scaffold ligaments of the breast

Cooper's ligament of the inguinal canal AKA – Pectineal ligament

Cooper's ligament of the elbow – transverse fibres of the ulnar collateral ligament

Denonvilliers' fascia – Rectoprostatic fascia

Douglas' line AKA The arcuate line of the abdomen AKA linea semicircularis – inferior border of the posterior layer of the rectus sheath. Point at which the inferior epigastric vessels perforate the rectus abdominis muscle

Drummond (Marginal Artery) – arterial arcade of the colon from the confluence of the SMA and IMA. Regarding the IMA, the Drummond artery is Distal and the arc of Riolan is proximally in relation to the root of the mesentery.

Dentate line AKA Pectinate line – Border between upper 2/3 and lower 1/3 of the anal canal at the hindgut-proctodeum junction

Erb's point (in the neck) – location at the posterior border of the sternocleidomastoid muscle where four superficial branches of the cervical plexus emerge: (1)greater auricular nerve, (2)lesser occipital nerve, (3)transverse cervical nerve, and (4)supraclavicular nerve (see Erb's auscultation point on the praecordium)

Galen (vein) AKA Vena Magna Galeni – Persistent thymic vein which can ocassionally be a source of superior mediastinal widening in newborns, infants and young children. Not to be confused with the vein of Galen in the brain AKA Vena Magna Cerebri Galeni AKA Great Cerebral Vein and also the internal cerebral veins (deep cerebral veins)

Gastric Anatomy:

Vagus: Left – Anterior, Right – Posterior

Left Vagus (anterior)→ Hepatic Branch →Gives off Branch to Pylorus

Left Vagus (anterior)→ Stomach Branches →Gives off Latarjet Nerve to Pylorus

Posterior Trunk Branch – Criminal nerve of Grassi, passes to the left posterior to the oesophagus and supplies the cardia of the stomach

Anterior Trunk Branch – Nerve of Latarjet supplying the

pylorus

Crow's foot – fanning out of Laterjet nerves

Latarjet Sparring Vagotomy AKA Highly selective vagotomy (HSV) AKA parietal cell vagotomy – targeting gastric, non-Laterjet branches of the gastric vagus branches to decrease acid release but preserve pyloric function

Truncal Vagotomy – transection vagal trunks requiring pyloroplasty as pyloric clearance decreased

Latarjet inclusive vagotomy AKA Selective Vagotomy (SV) – transection of the anterior and posterior Latarjet nerves below coeliac (right/posterior) and hepatic (left/anterior). This requires pyloroplasty as pyloric clearance is decreased.

Glisson's capsule AKA Liver capsule – Connective tissue encasing the liver, hepatic artery, portal vein, and bile ducts

Gerota's Fascia – Fibrous fascia encapsulating the kidneys and the adrenal glands

Grynfeltt-Lesshaft triangle AKA Superior lumbar triangle – (floor) transversalis fascia, (medial) quadratus lumborum muscle, (lateral) internal oblique, (superior) twelfth rib, (roof) external oblique

Hartmann's pouch – Junction between gallbladder neck and cystic duct

Hilton's white line AKA pecten of Robert Austin Stroud AKA Intersphincteric groove of the anus – anal transition line from non-keratinized stratified squamous epithelium to keratinized stratified squamous epithelium (leading to peri-anal skin). Below this line the lymphatic drainage drains to the superficial inguinal nodes

His (Angle of) – Angle between the stomach cardiac and the lower oesophagus

Hunter's canal AKA subsartorial canal AKA Adductor canal – aponeurotic tunnel connecting the femoral triangle at its apex to the adductor hiatus to allow the femoral vessels from the anterior thigh to the posterior thigh on to the popliteal fossa

Keynes (Great vein of) – Posterior venous drainage of the thymus gland

Kerckring folds AKA plicae circulares – valvulae conniventes

Kuntz (nerve) – rare intrathoracic sympathetic chain variation where there is an intrathoracic ramus connecting the ventral ramus of the 1st thoracic nerve to the 2nd intercostal nerve. This takes place upstream of the point where the 1st thoracic nerve gives a branch to the brachial plexus

Morgagni (Hydatid of) AKA Appendix testis – Vestigial remnant of the Müllerian duct, torsion of this presents clinically with upper testicular pole pain and a blue spot on transillumination

Morrison's pouch AKA hepatorenal pouch – potential space between the liver and the right kidney

Mayo (Vein of) – Identifies the pylorus of the stomach

Oddi Sphincter AKA Sphincter of Oddi AKA Hepatopancreatic Sphincter AKA Glisson's sphincter –

muscular valve regulating bile and pancreatic fluid to the through the ampulla of Vater and thence onward into the duodenum (2nd part)

Petit triangle AKA Inferior lumbar triangle – (anterior) external oblique, (posterior) latissimus dorsi, (base) iliac crest

Peyer's patches – lymphoid nodules or lymph tissue associated with the small bowel

Radix mesenterii – base of the mesentery of the small bowel

Riolan (arc of) AKA AOR AKA Arc of Riolan AKA mesenteric meandering artery of Moskowitz AKA central anastomotic mesenteric arter – arterial arcade at confluence of IMA and SMA

Retroperitoneal organs – '**ROCK PADS**'

- **R**ectum
- **O**esophagus
- **C**olon (ascending and descending)
- **K**idneys and Ureters
- **P**ancreas (not tail)
- **A**orta and IVC
- **D**uodenum (2nd and 3rd Parts)
- **S**upra-renal/ adrenal gland

Santorini duct – accessory pancreatic duct (see Wirsung duct)

Scarpa's Fascia – Deeper (to Camper's Fascia) membranous layer (stratum membranosum) of the superficial fascia of the abdomen

Sibson's fascia – Suprapleural membrane

Traube's (semilunar/ crescent) space for spleen percussion – surface markings (1) superiorly, left sixth rib, (2) left mid-axillary line laterally, (3) left costal margin inferiorly corresponding to (a) left costal margin, (b) lower edge of the left lung, (c) anterior border of the spleen, the left costal margin and (d) left liver lobe inferior margin.

Treves' fold AKA 'bloodless fold of Treves' AKA iliocaecal veil/ ligament – illiocaecal fold of peritoneum and the junction of the ileum and vermiform appendix

White line of Toldt – Lateral reflection of posterior parietal peritoneum covering the mesentery of the ascending and descending colon

Winslow epiploic foramen boundaries – (superior) Caudate lobe, (inferior) first part of duodenum, (anterior) lesser omentum and portal triad (CBD, portal vein, common hepatic artery), (posteriorly) IVC

Wirsung duct – Pancreatic duct (see Santorini duct)

2.   ABDOMINAL EXAM

Blumberg's sign AKA rebound tenderness – In abdominal pain, during palpation pain is exacerbated by sudden release of palpation pressure, suggesting peritonism

Carnett's sign – In abdominal pain it differentiates abdominal wall from acute abdominal (peritoneal) pain. Positive test (e.g. rectus sheath haemtoma, hernia etc.) is if pain increases or remains unchanged with tensing of the abdominal wall (raising legs and extending neck). Negative test (e.g.peritonitis) is if pain decreases when the patient relaxes abdominal wall.

Castell's sign of splenomegaly – Percussion sign of change from resonance in full inspiration to dull on full expiration at eighth or ninth intercostal space at the left axillary line (Castell's point)

Fothergill's sign – If an anterior abdominal wall mass does move with flexion of the rectus muscles and does not cross the midline, it has a high probability of being a rectus sheath hematoma.

Markle's sign – peritoneal pain on shaking the abdomen or support on which it rests, e.g. bed, patients limb (foot or hip)

Nixon's sign for splenomegaly – whilst in right decubitus, percussion mid left costal margin and downward, if dullness beyond 8cm then the sign is positive

3.   APPENDICITIS

Aaron's sign – epigastric referred pain with McBurney's point pressure

Alder's sign AKA Klein's sign – If maximal point of right iliac fossa (RIF) tenderness when supine shifts on rolling on the left lateral side, then it is more likely that the pain is gynaecological in origin

Alvarado score AKA MANTRELS score – MANTRELS is a pneumonic for the score: Migration to the right iliac fossa, Anorexia, Nausea/Vomiting, Tenderness in the right iliac fossa, Rebound pain, Elevated temperature (fever), Leukocytosis, and Shift of neutrophils to the left or neutrophilia. The modified Alvarado score is known by the pneumonic as MAFLTRN - My Appendix Feels Likely To Rupture Now

Arapov's sign (contracture) – reflex right hip contraction

Aure-Rozanova's sign of a retroceacal appendix AKA Shchetkin-Boomberg's sign – pain on palpation of the right Petit (lumbar) triangle

Dieulafoy's triad – McBurney's point (1) guarding, (2) skin hyperaesthesia and (3) Severe pain

Dunphy's sign – RIF pain on coughing

Markle sign AKA jar landing tenderness – Ball of foot standing to heel drop causing RIF pain

Massouh sign – Facial grimace following anterior abdominal finger sweep to the right (and not left). The sweep follows a path from xiphisternum to right iliac fossa (RIF) and left iliac fossa (LIF) respectively

Murphy's triad – (Pain → Vomiting → Fever), originally described as four signs (Abdominal pain → Vomiting → Right sided abdominal sensitiveness → Temperature)

McBurney's point – 2/3 of distance between umbilicus and anterior superior iliac spine

Ochsner-Sherren regimen – expectant management of appendix mass, that traditionally was followed by interval appendicectomy although more recently an interval procedure may not be necessary if the original inflammatory episode settles

Psoas sign – extending hip with knee fully extended to illicit pain

Rogozov appendicectomy AKA Cosmonaut appendicectomy – (i) auto-appendicectomy (done on oneself) and (ii) prophylactic appendicectomy before travelling to harsh environments such as Space or the Antarctic

Rosenstein's sign AKA Sitkovskiy sign – Pain exacerbation on moving from supine to recumbent

Rovsing's sign – LIF (left iliac fossa) palpation leading to RIF pain

Semm appendicectomy – Laparoscopic approach

Sherren's triangle – Hyperaesthesia between anterior superior iliac spine, the pubic tubercle and umbilicus

Appendicectomy incisions

Incisions: (Over McBurney's point 2/3 along line starting at umbilicus and ending at anterior superior iliac spine)

Lanz – along Langer's lines

McBurney – AKA Gridiron incision (oblique cut)

Rocky-Davis – Horizontal

Fowler-Weir – medial extension with medial cutting over the rectus

Rutherford-Morrison – lateral extension of McBurney (in hockey stick fashion) lateral and upward, muscle cutting internal oblique and transversus abdominis. Used also for access to the retroperitoneum

4. BARIATRIC

Buchwald-Varco operation – Partial Ileal Bypass

DeMeester Duodenal Switch procedure – non-bariatric, non-bypass procedure for the management biliary reflux gastritis

Dyspnea scales – Baseline Dyspnea Index (BDI), Borg (modified), cardiopulmonary exercise test, CPX, 6-min walking test, 6MWT, CR 10 (10 Category-Ratio), Rating of Perceived Exertion (RPE), Transitional Dyspnea Index (TDI), Visual Analogue Scale (VAS)

Fobi operation AKA Capella procedure AKA Fobi-Capella Bypass AKA Banded Gastric Bypass – Modification of the Banded Pouch Roux-en-Y Gastric Bypass

Hess Duodenal Switch AKA Hess-Scopinaro procedure AKA Biliopancreatic Diversion with Duodenal Switch (BPD-DS) – metabolic, malabsorptive bypass procedure where biliopancreatic fluid remains far upstream of food in the alimentary limb of a bypass construction

Huber needle – needle with specialised bevel to empty and drain fluid in gastric band ports

Internal Herniation Signs: (i) Whirl sign, (ii) internal hernia fluid in remnant, (iii) mushroom sign, (iv) clustered loops, (v) bowel behind SMA, (vi) right-sided J-J, (vii) hurricane eye, (viii) distended small bowel sign

Laidlaw disease AKA nesidioblastosis – Pancreatic Beta-cell hyperplasia from the Greek 'nesidioblast' or islet builder, can result in hyperinsulinaemic hypoglucaemia after bypass procedures

Magenstrasse – german for stomach road, lesser curve route for gastric contents from fundus to duodenum in 10minutes

Mason-Ito I Operation AKA Roux-en-Y Gastric Bypass

Mason-Ito II Operation AKA Gastrectomy and loop gastroenterostomy (gastrojejunostomy)

Mason Gastroplasty – Vertical Banded Gastroplasty

Hess Procedure AKA Hess-Marceau procedure – Biliopancreatic diversion with duodenal switch

Hertz syndrome AKA dumping syndrome – postprandial symptoms due to rapid
gastric drainage after gastroenterostomy. Two types: (1) Early immediately to <30mins after a meal, Abdominal pain, Dizziness, Palpitations, Dizziness, Hypotension likely due to foregut vagal signalling (2) Late 1-3hours Fatigue, Hunger, Perspiration, Tremor likely due to insulin, hypoglycaemia, gut hormone/incretin effects +/- vagal effects

Kremin-Linner-Nelson (first) – Jejunoileal Bypass

Lockwood Abdominoplasty – High-lateral-tension abdominoplasty

Magenstrasse and Mill gastroplasty – Forerunner to sleeve gastrectomy

O-sign – of gastric band, represents a coronal band looking like an 'o' on x-ray representing a slipped band (see Phi angle)

Pars flaccida AKA caudal hepatogastric ligament or gastrohepatic ligament

Payne procedure – Jejunoileal bypass

Pitanguy procedure – Abdominal lipectomy

Phi angle – 30-60 degree angle of appropriately placed gastric band, when beyond this angle on X-rays, it may represent a slip

Petersen space space/hernia – Iatrogenic internal space/hernias after Roux-en-Y Gastro-jejunostomy or Duodeno-jejunostomy between the transverse mesocolon and the meso-ileum (mesentry of the small bowel) of gastro-jejunostomy (or duodeno-jejunostomy) loop, and the retroperitoneum

Quetelet index AKA BMI AKA Body Mass Index – weight(kg)/height^2 (m^2)

Ramirez abdominoplasty – consists of making a longitudinal external oblique aponeurosis incision 1–2cm from the outer rectus abdominis border

Regnault prodecure – W-abdominoplasty

Refeeding syndrome – introduction of nutrition to a severely malnourished/ starved patient resulting in electrolyte imbalance (specifically hypophosphataemia and subsequent cardiac, CNS and respiratory patholohgy and symptoms

Roux-en-O – Iatrogenic morphology where the biliopancreatic limb of an RYGB anastomosed to the stomach pouch to create a closed loop-O

Roux-en-Y AKA Cesar Roux-en-Y AKA Ansa-en-Y anastomosis – Y-shaped bowel or bowel-stomach anastomosis, initially designed to prevent bile reflux (though now has multiple autobionic properties)

Roux-limb – alimentary limb of Roux-en-Y Gastric Bypass

Sarr operation AKA Henle limb procedure – procedure to reverse post RYGB hypoglycaemia by shortening the Y configuration

Schauer cap – omentum to protect Gastrojejunal anastomosis at Roux-en-Y Gastric Bypass

Sellick manoeuvre – cricoid pressure, used whilst administering methylene blue when test for a leak

Scopinaro operation AKA Biliopancreatic diversion

Scott procedure – Jejunoileal bypass

STOP BANG – Acronymous score for Obstructive Sleep Apnea: Snoring, Tiredness, Observed apnea, blood Pressure, Body mass index, Age, Neck circumference and Gender.

Torres operation AKA SADI-S procedure – SADI Single Anastomosis Duodenoileal bypass

Tumescent Liposuction AKA Klein liposuction

Wernicke's encephalopathy AKA Wernicke's disease – Neurological symptoms associated with B-vitamin deficiency (particularly thiamine-B1), associated with the triad of ophthalmoplegia, ataxia, and confusion

Wernicke–Korsakoff syndrome – concurrent existence of Wernicke's encephalopathy (WE) and Korsakoff's syndrome due to thiamine-B1 deficiency. Presenting with Wernicke's encephalopathy triad (see above) and Korsakoff syndrome (anterograde amnesia, variable presentation of retrograde amnesia and one of: Aphasia, Apraxia, Agnosia and a deficit in executive functions)

5. BASIC BIOCHEMISTRY AND PHYSIOLOGY

Anrep effect –autoregulation of myocardial contractility

Barr body – on X chromosomes when they are inactive, e.g. XXY Klinefelter's syndrome or XXXY

Bowditch effect AKA Treppe phenomenon AKA Treppe effect AKA Staircase effect – autoregulation of myocardial tension to increases concomitant to heart rate

Bowman's capsule – location where glomerular filtration occurs. Of note **ABCHDD** of renal physiology

A-Afferent arteriole (inflow of blood)
B-Bowman's capsule (glomerular filtration)
C-Proximal Convoluted Tubule (95% of glucose reabsorbed here)
H-Henle loop (with vasa recta, Water leaves Descending limb by diffusion due to potential created by Ascending Limb actively transporting of sodium and chloride), Frusemide acts here

D-Distal convoluted tubule (location of macula densa [part of juxtaglomerular apparatus, other being jxtg cells in arterioles and extraglomerular mesangial cells], sitting at hilum of B-Bowman's capsule, they are sensitive to blood flow and NaCl setting off RAAS system - renin–angiotensin–aldosterone system. Aldosterone works here), Thiazides act here

D-Duct(collecting duct, electrolyte homeostasis and ADH functioning through aquaporins)

Contraction alkalosis – raised blood pH due to fluid loss/ volume contraction (usually in severe vomiting). Renin-angiotensin pathway activated, resulting in aldosterone release and favouring of H+ loss over Na+ retention. Additionally, hypokalaemia and raised bicarbonate.

Coombs and Gell classification of Hypersensitivity – ACIDAR types:

I-A-Allergy/ Atopy, IgE

II-C-Cytotoxic antibody, IgM, IgG, Complement, MAC, Goodpasture Syndrome, Haemolytic anaemia, Rheumatic heart diease

III-I-Immune Complex, IgG, Complement, Neutrophils, serum sickness, Arthus reaction, SLE, RA

IV-D-Delayed Hypersensitivity/ cell-mediated, T-cells, Transplant rejection, Hashimoto's

V-AR-Autoimmune receptor (sometimes considered as type II), IgM, IgG, Complement, Graves', Myasthaenia Gravis

Cuthbertson Classification of Trauma Metabolism – (1) Ebb, Non-esterified fatty acid usage, 24-48 HOURS [ACUTE] (2) Flow, Loss of Nitrogen (Catabolic phase) 3-10 DAYS [CHRONIC], (3) Recovery, nitrogen levels increase (Anabolic phase) [WEEKS]. If failure to recover then anaerobic metabolism, necrobiosis and death

Epstein-Barr virus (EBV) – dsDNA Herpesviridae virus

Fluids

70kg man
water 60% (42L)

EI-EI-IT with all the branching at the 'E's'
1st E's cellular
2nd E's vascular

E(Extracellular 1/3 – 14L) + I(Intracellular 2/3 – 28L)
   ↓
E(Extravascular 11L) + I(Intravascular 3L Plasma)
   ↓
I(Interstitial 10.5) + T(Transcellular 0.5L)

Hartmann's solution AKA Ringer's lactate solution AKA sodium lactate solution (note: different Hartmann to that of Hartmann's operation and Hartmann's pouch). Note Hartman's solution and Ringer's lactate are not in fact identical. Hartmann's solution (units in mmol/L): Na131, K5, Cl111, Ca2, Lac29, Ringer's lactate: Na130, K4, Cl109, Ca1.5, Lac28. For comparison, 0.9% Normal saline: Na154, Cl154, 5% Dextrose only 50g/L of dextrose and 0.18%Dextrose saline only Na31 and 50g/L dextrose

von Gierke disease AKA Glycogen storage disease type I – genetic deficiency of the enzyme glucose-6-phosphatase, association with hepatic adenoma

Henderson–Hasselbalch equation – to calculate physiological pH

Hypo-Sal æratus-aemia AKA low bicarbonate levels – Hyperchloraemic Metabolic Acidosis – decreases anion gap. $H_2O + CO_2 \Leftrightarrow H_2CO_3 \Leftrightarrow H^+ + HCO_3^-$, in pancreatic fistula loss of HCO_3^- so hyperchloraemia predominates

Korotkoff sounds of blood pressure –

Phase I - First sound
Phase II - Whooshing
Phase III – Loud mid sound
Phase IV – Soft muffling
Phase V - Sound vanish completely at diastolic pressure

Kreb's Cycle AKA tricarboxylic acid cycle AKA citric acid cycle – generates energy in mitochondria by metabolising Acetyl CoA to $CO_2 + H^+$
Acetyl CoA (2C, comes from Pyruvate) +Oxaloacetate (4C)
Citrate (6C)
Isocitrate (6C)
Alpha-ketogultarate (5C) ***only 5C***
Succinyl-CoA (4C)
Succinate (4C)
Fumarate (4C)
Malate (4C)
Oxaloacetate (4C)

Oat Cell Cancer – Lung Cancer Type associated with SIADH (Syndrome of inappropriate ADH; also other drugs e.g. carbamazepine, SSRI's tumour, injury etc..)

Paul Bunnell test – for glandular fever

Sarnoff and Berglund curve – updated Starling curve explaining the Law of the Heart and cardiac output

Starling curve – mathematical description of cardiac output regulation

Stewart Acid-Base Technique – to calculate physiological pH

Warburg effect – Cancer cells tend to favour anaerobic Glycolysis for metabolism

Warburg hypothesis – Based on analysing the Warburg effect, where cancer growth may outstrip aerobic energy sources and therefore anaerobic glycolysis is utilised to fill this energy gap which essence becomes the driver of tumourigenesis

6. BREAST

Adams reconstruction AKA Nipple reconstruction. Multiple modern variations including fishtail flap, bow-and-arrow flap, star flap, skate flap, arrow flap, tab flap, S-flap, C-V flap, cylindrical flap, H-flap and pinwheel flap

Allred score – sensitivity of a breast tumour to oestrogens (oestrogen receptor status), utilising immunohistochemistry for oestrogen receptor (ER) (0 to 5) and the intensity of that staining (0 to 3), with a maximum score of 8

ANDI (Aberations in the Normal Development and Involution of the breast) – classification of benign breast disease: (a) disorders of development, (b) disorders of cyclical change, (c) disorders of involution

Baker classification of capsular contracture – (I) breast looks and feels normal. (II) minimal contracture that is clinically discernable but with no symptoms. (III) moderate contracture with patient experiencing symptoms of firmness. (IV) Severe, readily noticeable and clearly symptomatic contracture

BIRADS – Breast Imaging-Reporting and Data System. 0-incomplete, I-Negative, II-benign, III-probably benign, IV-suspicious of malignancy, V-highly suggestive of malignancy, VI-biopsy proven malignancy

Breast mouse – Fibroadenoma

Comedo AKA comedo necrosis AKA plug necrosis AKA Grade III DCIS – High-grade DCIS with histological presence of a 'plug'. Other types of DCIS (grades I [low grade] and II [moderate grade]) include Solid DCIS, Papillary DCIS and Cribriform DCIS AKA Swiss cheese DCIS. Of note Atypical ductal hyperplasia (ADH) shares some histological features of DCIS, and sometimes they are only distinguished by numbers of ducts involved

Cobblestoning AKA Fibrocystic breast AKA Benign mammary dysplasia – benign breast conditon

DIEP flap – Abdominal breast reconstruction technique utilising deep inferior epigastric perforators approach with skin and no muscle

Eggshell calcifications – mammographic finding of either fat necrosis or oil cysts (see also eggshell calcification in cardiac section)

Foote-Stewart disease AKA Foote-Stewart-Ewing disease – LCIS or lobular carcinoma in-situ

Grisotti flap – breast conserving technique utilised for reconstruction of central retroareolar breast cancers

Hadfield's procedure – radical subareolar duct excision, typically used to treat mammary duct fistulae

Hickmann line – Double lumen catheter, typically used

for chemotherapy

Halsted Mastectomy – Classical mastectomy procedure

Mastopexy (only breast skin)/ mammoplasty (breast tissue) modification of breast ptosis/sagging types:

Anchor AKA Lexer pattern
Wise/ Wyse/ Inverted T
Lollipop
J

Mondor's Disease – Superficial breast vein inflammation resulting to erythema and a prominent chord structure (vein)

Montgomery's Gland AKA Areolar glands – Prominent glands (secreting lubricating fluid) presenting as hard nodules on the peri-areolar area during breastfeeding

Nottingham Prognostic Index – I = (0.2 x Size[cm]) + Stage + Grade, score of predicted survival after breast surgery. 2-2.4 93%, >2.4-3.4 85%, >3.4-5.4 70%, >5.4 50%

Paget's Disease of the Breast– Eczema-like changes at the nipple associated with underlying cancer. There may be inversion, eversion and discharge due to retrograde extension of an intra-ductal carcinoma

Peau d'orange "orange skin" – Dimpled skin seen in inflammatory breast cancer

Phyllodes tumour AKA cystosarcoma phylloides – Rare, rapid growing, fibroepithelial breast tumours deriving from periductal stromal cells of the breast. Treated with Wide Local Excision and not sensitive to radio- or chemotherapy. From the Latin phyllodium and ancient Greek phullodes, to resemble a leaf

Radial scar AKA Complex sclerosing lesion – could be representative of Scirrhous carcinoma or Atypical ductal hyperplasia

Scirrhous carcinoma – sub-type of invasive ductal carcinoma

TRAM flap – Abdominal breast reconstruction technique utilising a Transverse Rectus Abdominis Myocutaneous flap

Triple investigation rule –
Mammography sensitivity 70-90%, specificity 75-95%
MRI sensitivity 95%, specificity 65%
Ultrasound sensitivity 85%, specificity 50-65%
Palpation sensitivity 50%, specificity 70-90%
Cytology sensitivity 90-95%, specificity 95%

Van Nuys – prognostic index for ductal carcinoma in situ (DCIS)

V-Y plasty – utilised to cover defects and wounds in breast surgery, but also a technique utilised for reconstructive surgery in general

Velpeau disease – Galactocoele

Viridi caseus AKA Green cheese discharge – sign of Duct Ectasia

Winging Scapula – Long Thoracic Nerve of Bell injury (C5-C7), also Thoracodorsal to LD results in weakness of abduction and intercostobrachial results in paraesthesia of upper inner arm

7. CARDIAC AND THORACIC

Bayford-Autenrieth dysphagia / syndrome AKA **Dysphagia lusoria** – Dysphagia due to aberrant right subclavian artery

Batista procedure AKA left ventriculoplasty AKA partial left ventriculectomy – aimed at minimising the wall tension (due to according to the LaPlace's law) in dilated cardiomyopathy

Blalock–Thomas–Taussig shunt AKA Blalock–Taussig shunt – surgical shunt created in cyanotic heart disease ('blue baby disease') connecting either (i) isolated subclavian artery or (ii) isolated carotid artery to the pulmonary artery. Used as a first stage to the Fontan procedure

Beck's triad of cardiac tamponade – (1) raised JVP or CVP, (2) reduced BP and (3) muffled heart sounds

Cutler procedure – closed mitral commisurotomy with cardiovalvulotome

David procedure AKA David-Feindel procedure (aortic)– Aortic Valve Sparring Root Replacement with coronary re-implantation

De Baillon disease AKA Empyema Necessitatis – Pleural empyema extending to the thoracic wall

Dotter technique AKA Dotter Gruentzig technique – originator of angioplasty and percutaneous intervention. Catheter clearance of obstructed vessel and subsequently dilatation of stenosis by dilators or balloon angioplasty

Eggshell calcification of lymph nodes – X-ray sign with multiple differentials, ranging from silicosis, lymphoma, sarcoidosis, amyloidosis, scleroderma, histoplasmosis, blastomycosis in addition to thymic cysts, aneurysms, pulmonary artery hypertension and parathyroid tumours

Elephant trunk technique – staged cardiovascular procedure where a graft placed at aortic arch/ root repair can be utilised for descending thoraco-abdominal aortic disease further down as a second stage

Erb's auscultation point (on the praecordium) – location on the S2 is best auscultated (3rd intercostal space [ICS] on the left sternal border). 2nd ICS on the right of the sternum=aortic, 2nd ICS on the left of the sternum=pulmonary, 4th ICS on the left of the sternum=tricuspid, 5th ICS on the left of the sternum=mitral (see Erb's point in the neck)

Fontan procedure AKA Fontan–Kreutzer procedure – applied for univentricular heart circulations (where the left side of the heart is under-developed), redirecting IVC and SVC directly to the pulmonary arteries (bypassing the right heart).

Glenn Shunt AKA bidirectional Glenn shunt AKA hemi-Fontan procedure – The superior vena cava redirected to drain into the right pulmonary artery

Good's syndrome – Acquired immunodeficiency (combined B and T cell) associated with thymoma. Important consideration during thymectomy due to increased susceptibility to infection

Hoffman-Rigler sign – x-ray identification of LV enlargement based on distance bwetween IVC and LV

Hassall's corpuscles AKA Thymic corpuscles bodies – Concentric thymic cells derived from eosinophilic type VI epithelial reticular cells, have a possible pathogenic role in several autoimmune diseases. Thymus itself is an anterior mediastinal lymphoid organ developing from the endoderm of the third pharyngeal pouch

Jatene procedure (transposition of the great arteries) – arterial switch procedure

Karoshi – Precipitous mortality/ collapse due to overwork

Kussmaul's (paradoxical) sign of cardiac tamponade – raised JVP or CVP on inspiration

ECG/EKG (electrocardiogram):

QT=typically Calcium levels, Cal_QT
QRS=typically Potassium Levels, Pot_QRS

J waves – Hypothermia

Prolonged QT – HypoCalcaemia, Romano-Ward syndrome, Jervell and Lange-Nielsen syndrome. Also hypokalaemia, hypomagnesemia

Short QT – HyperCalcaemia

Right axis deviation – Pulmonary Embolus (PE)
SI QIII TIII – Pulmonary Embolus (PE)
Right Bundle Branch Block – Pulmonary Embolus (PE)

T wave flattening/inversion – HypoKalaemia
U wave – HypoKalaemia
Apparent long QT – HyoKalaemia
Peaked T waves – HyperKalaemia

Widened QRS – HyperKalaemia

Favaloro operation – coronary artery bypass with reversed saphenous vein

Galavardin Phenomenon – Dissociation between the noisy and musical elements of the aortic stenosis murmur

Heyde's syndrome – gastrointestinal bleeding from angiodysplasia associated with aortic stenosis secondary to Von Willebrand factor (vWF) depletion as a result of altered blood flow through the stenosed aortic valve

Lecompte maneuver of arterial switch procedures – neo-aorta behind pulmonary artery bifurcation
Lutembacher Syndrome – congenital atrial septal defect (ASD) + acquired mitral stenosis

Marantic Endocarditis AKA Non-bacterial thrombotic endocarditis (NBTE)

Mustard procedure (transposition of the great arteries) – corrects transposition at the atrial level, resecting atrial septum, utilises artificial or pericardial patch/baffle to connect/ shunt systemic blood in the right ventricle to the left ventricle (similar to the Senning procedure)

Norwood procedure – used in Hypoplastic left heart syndrome, creating a neo-aorta from the pulmonary trunk

Ortner's syndrome (I) – left recurrent laryngeal nerve palsy from cardiovascular disease, typically the left atrial dilatation of mitral stenosis

Ortner's syndrome II – abdominal angina.

Pape dysphagia / syndrome AKA **Dysphagia aortica** – Dysphagia due to extrinsic oesophageal compression due to thoracic aortic aneurysm

Pancoast tumour AKA pulmonary sulcus tumour AKA superior sulcus tumour – pulmonary sulcus tumour typically causing Horner's syndrome (AKA Claude-Bernard-Horner syndrome)

Pancoast-Tobias syndrome – (1) Horner's syndrome (AKA Claude-Bernard-Horner syndrome), (2) shoulder pain radiating to the axilla or scapula (or both) and down the ulnar distribution of the upper limb, (3) hand and arm muscle atrophy (4) subclavian vein obstruction with upper arm oedema

Rastelli operation – Surgical patch for directing oxygenated blood from the left ventricle to aorta

Ross I Procedure – Pulmonary autograft to aortic position

Ross II Procedure AKA Ross-Kabani Procedure – Pulmonary autograft to mitral position

Senning procedure AKA 'two wrongs make a right' procedure (transposition of the great arteries) – utilises atrial septum as a patch/baffle to connect/ shunt systemic blood in the right ventricle to the left ventricle (similar to the Mustard procedure)

Souttar Procedure – closed mitral commisurotomy with finger dilatation

Takotsubo Syndrome AKA Takotsubo cardiomyopathy AKA Broken Heart Syndrome AKA Stress cardiomyopathy AKA Octopus trap syndrome – emotionally triggered sudden-onset non-ischaemic cardiomyopathy

Weinberg Operation – Implantation of internal mammary arteries into the myocardium

Yacoub procedure (aortic)– Aortic Valve Sparring Root Replacement with remodelling

Yacoub procedure (transposition of the great arteries) – two-stage arterial switch procedure

8. COLORECTAL CANCER AND PROCEDURES

Dukes staging system for colorectal cancer – predicts mortality based on histology:

Dukes A (T1N0M0 or T2N0M0): tumour within bowel wall, 90% 5 year survival

Dukes B (T3N0M0 or T4N0M0): Beyond bowel wall but without lymph node involvement, 70% 5 year survival)

Dukes C ([any T]N1M0 or [any T]N2M0): With lymph node involvement, 30% 5 year survival

Dukes D ([any T and N] M1): Metastases

Ferguson haemorrhoidectomy AKA closed haemorrhoidectomy

Gardner Syndrome AKA Gardner's Syndrome = FAP (familial adenomatous polyposis) + Benign Tumours + Malignant Tumour Risk. Mutation in the adenomatous polyposis coli (APC tumour suppressor gene) on chromosome 5q21 (band q21 on chromosome 5). Not related, but another inherited non-hamartomatous polyposis syndrome is MUTYH-associated polyposis AKA MYH-associated polyposis (MAP)

Benign = osteomas (usually skull and jaw), fibromas and sebaceous cysts, epidermoid cysts, desmoids

Malignant = Colonic (100%)+ Small bowel (4%-12%), Pancreatic (2%), Papillary thyroid (2%), Hepatoblastoma(1.5%) CNS(<1%), Stomach(0.5%) Biliary, Adrenal. In the duodenal FAP there is the Spigelman Classification of Duodenal Polyposis. Consists of: Number of polyps, Polyp size (mm), Histology, Dysplasia and Stage

Haggitt classification of Pedunculated Malignant Colorectal Polyps – Level 0 (in situ) to Level 4 (submucosa below stalk and above muscularis propria)

HALO procedure – Haemorrhoidal Artery Ligation Operation for haemorrhoids

Hartmann's Procedure AKA Proctosigmoidectomy – Proximal end of resection brought out at stoma

Heald 'holy plane' approach – Total Mesorectal Excision

Kikuchi classification of Sessile Polyps AKA Kudo level (and not Kudo classification) – Histological classification of colorectal polyp invasion into the submucosa, (1) Sm1 first third (2) Sm2 middle third (3) Sm3 lower third

Kraske operations – typically performed in Kraske's position (please see blow) where the coccyx and left sacrum are excised for access to rectal lesions. Can be performed by utilising Kraske's parasacral approach.

Kraske position – prone with flexed hips and forming a peak with both head and feet facing down, allows good exposure to the sacrum, coccyx and anorectal region (please see Kraske operation above)

Lynch syndrome = HNPCC (Hereditary nonpolyposis colorectal cancer)

These are due to DNA mismatch repair defects due to MSI-H (MSI, MicroSatellite Instability) affecting MLH1 and MSH2 tumour suppressor genes

Lynch syndrome I (familial colon cancer, i.e. 'pure' HNPCC of the colon)

Lynch syndrome II (HNPCC + cancers of the gastrointestinal tract or reproductive system)

Lynch syndrome criteria – (a) Amsterdam/Amsterdam II AKA '3-2-1' criteria: 3 or more relatives with an associated cancer; 2 or more successive generations affected; 1 or more relatives diagnosed before the age of 50 years (1 should be a first-degree relative) (b) Bethesda criteria: Colorectal carcinoma (CRC) diagnosed <50 yr; Synchronous or metachronous Lynch syndrome-associated tumours; CRC with high microsatellite instability; CRC diagnosed in 1+ first-degree relatives with a Lynch syndrome-associated tumour <50yr; CRC diagnosed in 2+ first-degree or second-degree relatives with Lynch syndrome-associated tumours, regardless of age

Luschka's law – The Right ureter usually crosses the external iliac artery and the Left ureter crosses the common iliac artery (typically near the bifurcation)

McColl syndrome AKA – Juvenile polyposis syndrome with hamartomas in GI tract associated with mutations in

BMPR1A or SMAD4

Miles procedure AKA Traditional Abdominoperineal resection resection

Milligan-Morgan haemorrhoidectomy AKA Open haemorrhoidectomy

Muir-Torre Syndrome (? Lynch syndrome III)– HNPCC (Lynch I) + skin epitheliomas, epidermoid cysts, carcinoma, keratocanthoma, autosomal dominant

Paris endoscopic classification of superficial neoplastic lesions (oesophagus, stomach, and colon) – (see Japan classification in Gastric Cancer section)

Paul-Mikulikcz stoma – Two ends brought out, approximated and adjacent mucosal surfaces sutured

Peutz-Jeghers Syndrome (autosomal dominant) – Multiple gastrointestinal polyps (Hamartomatous) + mucocutaneous pigmentations (melanosis). Due to mutation in serine/threonine 11 gene (STK11). Risk of GI, Breast, ovary, uterus, testicular and pancreatic cancer and intussusception. Related to other Hamartomatous conditions, these include PTEN (gene mutation) hamartoma tumour syndromes: Cowden syndrome (hamartomatous intestinal polyposis + multiple tricholemmomas) and follicular thyroid cancer AKA COLD syndrome (acronym) for Cowden + Lhermitte-Duclos disease, now considered a phakomatosis (neurocutaneous embryonic ectoderm condition), Bannayan-Zonana syndrome AKA Bannayan-Riley-Ruvalcaba syndrome, Lhermitte-Duclos disease (AKA Dysplastic Gangliocytoma of the Cerebellum), Proteus syndrome AKA Wiedemann syndrome, Proteus-like syndrome and juvenile polyposis syndrome. See above,

McColl syndrome, Juvenile polyposis syndrome with hamartomas, mutations in BMPR1A or SMAD4

Quirke protocol – Margins in Colorectal Cancer

Sugarbaker technique – Complete cytoreduction for pseudomyxoma peritonei

Turnbull-Cutait abdominoperineal pull-through – designed to prevent permanent diversion in patients with complex anorectal conditions

Typhilitis AKA Caecitis AKA Neutropaenic enterocolitis – Caecal inflammation possibly leading to necrosis, sometimes seen after administration of cytotoxic chemotherapy (Not the same as CMV colitis which can be seen in immunocompromised patients diagnosed antigen status, serology colonoscopic biopsy)

Whitehead's circumferential radical haemorroidectomy – Utilises modified sliding skin-flap grafts

9.   COLORECTAL (BENIGN)

Fistulas

Goodsall's law – fistulas with anterior external opening (anterior to the transverse midline) have a direct route to the anus, posterior one's take a non-straight or curved route

Rojanasakul procedure AKA LIFT technique – intersphincteric plane approach for fistula-in-ano (ligation of intersphincteric fistula tract)

Park's classification – Inter-, Trans-, Supra- and Extra-sphincteric

Colorectal Diseases

Bristol stool score – Liquidity of stool

Cleveland Clinic score – Faecal incontinence (i)frequency of incontinence to gas, (ii)liquid, (iii) solid matter, (iv)use of pads, (v)effect on daily lifestyle. Each variable scored 0-4 with a maximum of 20. (See also St Mark's score)

Coffee bean sign – radiological sign of sigmoid volvulus Also with barium enema, or contrast study, "Bird of Prey' sign

Crohn's Disease AKA Crohn-Ginzburg-Oppenheimer Disease – chronic inflammatory GI condition where there are (1) GI manifestations(bowel frequency, diarrhoea, aphthous ulcers and perianal fistulae) (2) Non-GI or extra-intestinal manifestations (skin [erythema nodosum, pyoderma gangrenosum], uveitis, episcleritis, spondyloarthritis, clubbing) manifestations. Histologically: can occur any part of GI tract, crypt abscesses, skip lesions, granulomas, transmural inflammation and fissures. SCUF

Skip lesions
Cobblestoning
Non-caseating granulomas
Lymphocytic infiltrates and lymphoid aggregates
Ulcers (deep and serpiginous)
Fissures (transverse)
Preservation of crypt architecture
Giant cells
NOT typically crypt abscesses

Crohn's = Cobbleski: Cobblestoning, Skip lesions, Ulcers, fissures

'Lead pipe' appearance on abdominal radiographs (due to loss of haustral fold pattern), also seen in ulcerative colitis

Also in Crohn's: Lockwood's sign AKA chronic appendicitis sign, palpation of peristalsis of air (flatulence) at McBurney's point

Strictuloplasty procedures for Crohn's include – (1) 'simple' **The Heineke-Mikulicz**, (2) 'intermediate' Finney, (3) 'complex' the Michelassi

Koch pouch AKA Continent Ileostomy – predecessor of the Nicholson ileoanal pouch (see below), consisting of a ileal S pouch (acting as a reservoir) with a one-way valve, so that the pouch can be emptied by the patient preference

Fournier's gangrene – Necrotising fasciitis of the perineum

Hinchey classification of Diverticulitis –
(I): localised abscess (para-colonic)
(II): pelvic abscess
(III): purulent peritonitis
(IV): faeculent peritonitis

Nicholson procedure AKA Restorative proctocolectomy with an ileoanal pouch – J-pouch (also W-pouch and S-pouch). See also Koch pouch above

Ogilvie syndrome – Colonic / intestinal pseudo-obstruction

Pilonidal Sinus Procedures – (1) Bascom Procedure AKA 'cleft lift procedure AKA 'cleft closure' procedure using the 'stay out of the ditch' philosophy, sinus excised by para-vertebral incision, (2) Karydakis AKA The modified Karydakis-Limberg Flap procedure for sacrococcygeal pilonidal sinus disease (SPSD), (3) Marsupialization technique

Rectal procidentia AKA Rectal prolapse – Eponymous operations

(i) Perineal: Delorme procedure (sleeve resection of

mucosa and rectal muscular plication), Altemeier perineal (proctosigmoidectomy with transanal proctectomy and colo-anal anastomosis), Parks (posterior anal repair), Thiersch (Perineal sling), Thomas (Suture rectopexy)

(ii) Anterior fixation: Ripstein rectopexy (anterior sling rectopexy, historically with Teflon), Pemberton (Sigmoidopexy), Nigro (Ventral Teflon sling)

(iii) Posterior fixation: Wells (posterior sling rectopexy, historically with an ivalon sling), Sudeck (Suture rectopexy)

(iv) Pelvic floor reconstruction: Moschcowitz (Douglas closure), Graham (Anterior levatoropexy), Goligher (Anterior + posterior levatoropexy), Sullivan (Total pelvic mesh repair)

(v) Formal Resection: Muir (Anterior resection), Frykman (Sigmoid resection + rectopexy)

Rome III Diagnostic Criteria for Functional Gastrointestinal Disorders

Stapled Transanal Rectal Resection (STARR) – For Obstructive Defecation Syndrome (ODS) and Rectocoele

Solitary rectal ulcer syndrome AKA ulcerative proctocolitis

St Mark's score – Faecal incontinence (See also Cleveland Clinic score)

St Mark's solution – glucose-electrolyte solution used in the management of short bowel syndrome

Thaysen disease AKA Proctalgia fugax – intermittent rectal pain with no identifiable pathology on investigations

Ulcerative Colitis – Chronic, relapsing inflammatory disease of the colon (anywhere from cecum to rectum); rarely exhibits peri-anal disease and 'backwash ileitis'. Histologically: crypt architecture changes (shortening and branching), crypt abscesses, inflammation usually confined to the mucosa and submucosa, goblet cell depletion, general inflammatory invasion. Unlike Crohn's, rare to find granulomas, transmural inflammation and serositis (except in toxic mega-colon). Pseudopolyps and dysplasia as a prelude to cancer can be present. Thickened muscularis mucosae, and also Paneth cell metaplasia. Bowel 'thumb printing' on x-ray die to mucosal oedema. 'Lead pipe' appearance on abdominal radiographs (due to loss of haustral fold pattern), also seen in Crohn's disease. Extraintestinal manifestations more common In UC than Crohn's and include pyoderma gangrenosum, sclerosing cholangitis, ankylosing spondylitis and chronic active hepatitis. Much higher risk for colon cancer. 10% of patients with IBD not UC or Crohn's so called indeterminate colitis

UC Histology = PsuedoCryptic: Crypt abscesses, Pseudopolyps, Mucosa-only

Mayo clinic score – UC severity score

Truelove and Witts' severity index – Classifies severity of Ulcerative Colitis as mild, moderate and severe comprising of: (1) Bowel movements, (2) stool blood, (3) Temperature, (4) Pulse, (5) Anaemia, (6) ESR

10. ENDOCRINE

Addison's disease – Adrenocortical deficiency (presentation includes hyperkalaemia[K+ ≥ 5.5 mmol/L] and hyponatraemia as there is impaired aldosterone release). Also acidosis and hypoglycaemia. Physiologically there is hypotension. Hyper K's: Kalaemia, Calcaemia, UriKaemia, (Hypos: Natraemia, Glycaemia, Hypotension)

Amiodarone Thyroid Effect AKA 'A-T3 or 83 Effect'– Hypothyroidism with normal T4 and low T3 (as peripheral conversion is affected, possibly through iodination or thyroiditis)

Becker syndrome AKA Glucagonoma – Presents with Necrolytic migratory erythema (NME) and Diabetes Mellitus

Berry's ligament AKA suspensory ligament of the thyroid gland – between thyroid sheath and thyroid onto cricoid cartilages

Berry's sign – Thyromegaly with absent or weak carotid pulse as the hypertrophied/malignant thyroid is encasing the carotid artery

Boettlin disease AKA Boettlin-Gottschalk-Von Kalden-

Wetteland Disease AKA Struma ovarii – thyroid teratoma of the ovary that can cause hyperthyroidism

Carney triad, subtype of multiple endocrine neoplasia (MEN) – (1) gastric GIST gastrointestinal stromal tumour (not c-kit associated although 80% of GISTs in general are), (2) Pulmonary chondroma, and (3) Extra-adrenal paraganglioma

Carney-Stratakis syndrome – (1) GIST and (2) Paraganglioma (mitochondrial tumour suppressor gene involving the succinate dehydrogenase subunits)

Carney Complex (unrelated to Carney Triad) AKA LAMB syndrome AKA NAME syndrome – (1) Myxomas of heart and skin (also neural and endocrine), (2) Skin hyperpigmentation (lentiginosis), (3) Endocrine over-activity

Cajal interstitial cell – origin cell of GISTs

Chvostek sign of hypocalcaemia – twitching of the facial muscles after facial nerve tap as a sign of hypocalcaemia (see Trousseau sign), also seen in hypomagnesaemia

Collar-stud abscess – tuberculous neck abscess, typically a 'cold-abscess' as no erythema (see also Ghon focus and Scrofula)

Conn's syndrome (adrenal adenoma) AKA primary hyperaldosteronism – Symptoms include fatigue, hypokalaemia, alkalosis, hypomagnesaemia, polyuria

Crowe sign AKA Crowe's sign – axillary (armpit) freckling associated with von Recklinghausen's disease (neurofibromatosis type I). Axillary freckling can also occur with Lynch syndrome/HNPCC and Legius syndrome (axillary freckling, cafe-au-lait spots), neurofibromas / CNS tumours, macrocephaly without Lisch nodules [i.e. without iris hamartomas]). May be associated with inguinal freckling in von Recklinghausen's disease (neurofibromatosis type I).

Cushing's Syndrome – Hypercortisolism, (1) Obesity (2) Fatty tissue deposits at the face [moon face], between shoulders [buffalo hump], midsection and upper back. (3) Purple or Pink stretch marks (striae) on the thorax, trunk or thighs (4) Echymoses (bruising) due to fragile and thining skin

Cushing's Disease – subset of Cushing's Syndrome, Hypercortisolism secondary to pituitary tumour secreting ACTH

Czyhlarz disease – Tracheomalacia, flaccidity of tracheal cartilage, rare but recognized complication after thyroidectomy

Delphian node – cervical lymph node (level VI) predictor of poor cancer outcome, named after the predictive capability of the ancient Oracle at Delphi

De Quervain's thyroiditis AKA subacute granulomatous thyroiditis AKA giant cell thyroiditis – typically viral in 20-50 year olds, can occur with pyrexia

Frey's syndrome AKA Baillarger's syndrome AKA Frey-Baillarger syndrome AKA Dupuy's syndrome AKA Gustatory neuralgia AKA Auriculotemporal syndrome –

parotid gland and auriculotemporal nerve damage during surgery resulting in gustatory cheek seating, and redness/ flushing

Gastrinoma Triangle – (1) confluence of cystic and hepatic duct, (2) junction of head and neck of pancreas, (3) junction between 2nd and 3rd part of duodenum

Graves' disease AKA toxic diffuse goitre – TSH receptor auto-antibodies. Goitre with bruit, dermopathy (Acropachy and pretibial myxoedema), and eye signs

Graves with eye signs is known as Graves-Basedow or Basedow-Graves-Parry-Flajani Disease. This may include congestive oculopathy demonstrated by chemosis (conjunctival swelling), conjunctivitis, periorbital oedema, corneal ulcers, optic nerve atrophy and optic neuritis. Eponymous signs include:

(1) Abadie's sign – Upper eyelid elevator weakness and dysfunction

(2) Boston's sign – Rapid upper eyelid closure on looking down

(3) Ballett's sign – loss of voluntary eyeball motion but pupillary reflexes remain

(4) Beck's sign – powerful pulsation of retinal arteries

(5) Coweh's sign – exaggerated pupillary constriction

(6) Darlymple's sign – widened eyelid opening and exposure of iris

(7) Enroth's sign – eyelid oedema (usually superior)

(8) Hertoghe's sign AKA Queen Anne's sign – lateral third eyebrow loss

(9) Gifford's sign – Jerky and laborious movement of superior eyelid

(10) Jellinek's sign – Hyperpigmented superior eyelid folds eyelids

(11) Jendrassik's sign – Limited abduction and rotation

due to paralysis of all extraocular muscles

(12) Joffroy's sign – loss of forehead crinkling on looking up

(13) Kocher's sign – loss of coordination between eyeballs and frontal muscles on upward gaze

(14) Loewi's sign – rapid adrenaline solution mydriasis

(15) Mann's sign – apparent incongruity of eye levels due to skin tanning/ bronzing

(16) Moebius sign – Squint and loss of convergence

(17) Movement's cap phenomenon – Jerky eyeball movements

(18) Rosenbach's sign – Superior eyelid tremor on closure

(19) Russel-Fraser's sign – Reduced fold angle between upper eyelid and eyeball on closure

(20) Saiton's sign – eyeball movement results in horizontal nystagmus

(21) Sattler's sign – elevated intraocular pressure

(22) Snellen-Rieseman's sign – Systolic bruit on auscultation of closed eyelid

(23) Stellwag's sign – extenuation of 'proptosis' status by upper eyelid retraction

(24) Suker's sign – difficulty in fixation on abduction

(25) Tellas's sign – Inferior eyelid pigmentation

(26) Topolanski's sign – vascular band and the four rectus muscle insertions

(27) Von Graefe's sign – loss of coordination between eyeball and superior eyelid on downward gaze

(28) Wilder's sign – apparent impression of rapid eyeball motion on sequential abduction and adduction

(29) Willbrand-Saenger's sign – augmented eyelid secretion to protect against failure to close eyelids (lagophthalmos)

Gluck-Sorenson incision AKA U-shaped flap (apron flap) incision for extensive neck surgery

Hamburger thyrotoxicosis – community thyroiditis as a result of eating beef contaminated with bovine thyroid tissue

Hashimoto's Thyroiditis AKA chronic lymphocytic thyroiditis – autoimmune thyroiditis with thyroid microsomal autoantibodies

Hürthle cell (adenoma and carcinoma) – associated with Hashimoto's thyroiditis and follicular thyroid cancer

Jod-Basedow effect – Hyperthyroidism secondary to high iodine intake (see also Wolff–Chaikoff effect)

Kocher incision AKA Collar incision – Horizontal incision for thyroidectomy

Ludwig's angina AKA Angina Ludovici AKA angina Maligna AKA Morbus Strangularis – infection (typically bilateral) at the fascial space of the submandibular, sublingual and submental glands, most commonly due to dental infections from alpha-haemolytic streptococci, staphylococci and bacteroides

Merlin gene disease AKA Neurofibromatosis type II AKA multiple inherited schwannomas, meningiomas, and ependymomas (MISME syndrome) – schwannomas with acoustic neuromas

Müller's muscle AKA Superior tarsal muscle – when inhibited by sympathetic nervous dysfunction can lead to the ptosis/ partial ptosis of Horner's syndrome

Nervus larygeus recurrens – supplies the posterior cricoarytenoid

Obendorfer disease AKA carcinoid syndrome AKA

Thorsen-Biorck-Björkman-Waldenstrom syndrome AKA Thorson-Bioerck syndrome AKA Cassidy-Scholte syndrome AKA Argentaffinoma syndrome AKA Flush syndrome – Neuroendocrine tumour of enterochromaffin cells (Kulchitsky cells) with gut hormone secretion, typically serotonin (5HT). Approximately 10% of carcinoids have the symptoms of carcinoid syndrome. These include:

(A) Abdominal pain (i.desmoplastic reaction of the mesentery ii.hepatic metastases)
(B) Bronchoconstriction (histamine-related)
(C) Cardiomyopathy (secondary restrictive type with endocardial fibrosis, TIPS-Tricuspid Insufficiency, Pulmonary Stenosis, when mitral valve involved typically results in a right-sided or pulmonary shunt)
(D) Diarrhoea
(E) Electrolyte disturbance
(F) Flushing
(G) GI symptoms (general, e.g. vomiting, nausea, cramps)
(H) Hepatomegaly

Diagnosis typically by 24-hour urine levels of 5-HIAA (5-hydroxyindoleacetic acid) as the end product of serotonin metabolism

Pak's classification of hypercalciuria – (i) absorptive hypercalciuria, (ii) renal hypercalciuria, (iii) resorptive hypercalciuria

Papillary Thyroid Cancer: Lymph Spread Follicular Thyroid Cancer: Blood Spread, may have Psammoma boies (see below)

Pick-Fränkel Disease – Phaeochromocytoma. Tested with 24hr urinary carecholamines and metanephrines (and plasma also) Treated initially with phenoxybenzamine then b-blocker in advance of surgery. Can also be tested with meta-iodo-benzyl-guanidine (MIBG) scan. Is associated with MEN II syndromes

Plummer's nail, onycholysis (nail separation from the nail bed) typically in the ring and little fingers in thyrotoxicosis

Potato tumours AKA Carotid Body Tumour AKA Chemodectoma – Painless and slow growing tumours that are rarely malignant. They can be pulsatile and present with transient cerebral ischaemia, blackout and occasionally vaso-vagals on examination

Psammoma body – 'sand-like', calcium collections, see in in Papillary cancers, typically Papillary thyroid carcinoma

Riedel's thyroiditis AKA Riedel's struma AKA Woody Thyroiditis – Chronic Thyroiditis with multi-system fibrotic involvement including the retroperitoneum

Salivary gland types – (i) Glands of Weber (pure mucous, lateral tongue border), (ii) Glands of von Ebner (pure serous) and (iii) Glands of Blandin and Nuhn (mixed mucous and serous glands)

Schmidt's syndrome – 2 of 3 of: Addison's disease, hypoparathyroidism, mucocutaneous candidiasis

Schwartz syndrome AKA Syndrome of inappropriate antidiuretic hormone secretion – hyponatraemia, low serum osmolality and high urine osmolality

Sistrunk procedure (different to Sistrunk procedure for lymphoedema) – Excision of thyroglossal cyst and/or sinus tract with concomitant excision of the hyoid bone

Sipple Syndrome (MEN IIA Syndrome, RET gene) – (1) Medullary Thyroid Carcinoma, (2) Phaeochromocytoma,

(3) Parathyroid Hyperplasia

Sizemore-Williams Syndrome AKA Wagenmann–Froboese syndrome AKA Williams-Pollock syndrome AKA Gorlin-Vickers syndrome (MEN II B Syndrome, RET gene) AKA 'MEN III though not common'– MEN II A + (1) Mucosal Neuromas (including intestinal ganglioneuromatosis), (2) Marfanoid Habitus and other symptoms, e.g. delayed puberty. Some people suggest lower prevalence of hyperparathyroidism in MEN II B

Thyroid nail disease – (Beau's lines see above), Hypothyroid Alunula (lack of the Lunula or nail-bed moon), Onychorrhexis (longitudinal nail-bed ridging), Onycholysis (longitudinal nail bed splitting)

Trousseau Disease AKA Trousseau-von Recklinghausen Disease AKA Haemochromatosis Type 1 AKA HFE gene Hereditary Haemochromatosis – iron overload condition due to genetic excessive absorption leading to classic triad of cirrhosis, bronze skin and diabetes but also systemic complaints of fatigue and impotence

Trousseau sign – sign of hypocalcaemia, caropedal spasm on inflating a blood-pressure cuff placed on the arm (see Chvostek sign), also seen in hypomagnesaemia

von Recklinghausen's Neurofibromatosis AKA morbus Recklinghausen – Neurofibromatosis I, mutation on chromosome 17. Lisch nodules (iris hamartomas), Crowe's sign (axillary freckling), café-au-lait spots AKA café au lait macules (CALMs), Lisch nodules (iris hamartomas), epilepsy, skin nodules (rubbery), scoliosis, learning disabilities, vision disorders, mental disabilities. Sometimes mistaken for Legius syndrome which also has café-au-lait spots

von Recklinghausen's disease – Osteitis Fibrosa Cystica with subperiosteal bone erosions associated with parathyroid adenoma

Waterhouse-Friderichsen syndrome – acute adrenal insufficiency secondary to bilateral intra-adrenal haemorrhage in patients associated with severe septicaemia (e.g. meningococcal). Can present with purpura, DIC, adrenal failure and rapid deterioration with multi-system failure and coma

Warthin's tumour AKA Papillary cystadenoma lymphomatosum – benign disease in smokers, typically aged 60-70yrs and bilateral in 5-14%

Willis- Frank syndrome AKA Diabetes Insipidus – too little ADH from the posterior pituitary, hypernatraemia, high serum osmolality, low urine osmolality. Two types: Neurogenic (e.g. brain injury) and Nephrogenic

Wermer Syndrome (MEN I Syndrome, MEN 1 gene) – (1) Pancreatic Tumour (e.g. gastrinoma and Zollinger–Ellison syndrome (ZES), insulinoma, glucagonoma), (2) Pituitary adenoma, (3) Parathyroid Hyperplasia

Whipple's Triad of Insulinomas – (1) Symptoms likely hypoglycemic in origin (e.g. fasting or exercise), (2) Symptoms coinciding with low plasma glucose, (3) Symptom relief on normalising glucose levels

Wolff–Chaikoff effect – Temporary hypothyroidism (7-10 days) secondary to intake of high amounts of iodine. Typically followed by an "escape phenomenon." This effect can be used to treat severe against hyperthyroidism, such as thyroid storm. (see also Jod-Basedow effect).

Zollinger-Ellison (Hypergastrinaemia) – (1) Peptic

ulcers and severe gastric acid release, (2) Diarrhoea, (3) Abdominal pain or triad of (i) Peptic ulceration (ii) Gastric acid hypersecretion, (iii) islet cell tumour of the pancreas (gastrinoma). Can be part of MEN 1 syndrome (see above)

Zuckerkandl (organ) – neural crest derived mass of chromaffin cells next to the aorta, starting above SMA or at renal arteries and extending to the aortic bifurcation, can be a non-adrenal site of Phaeocromocytomas (90% are adrenal). 10%extra-adrenal, 10%bilateral, 10% in children, 10% malignant and 10% multiple, treated by phenoxybenzamine

Zuckerkandl (tubercle) – non-pathological prominence on the posterior lateral thyroid gland (radiologically can sometimes be mistaken for a thyroid nodule). Lies on recurrent laryngeal nerve

11. GASTRIC CANCER

Borrmann classification of advanced gastric cancer – Type I: polypoid fungating, Type II: ulcerative with elevated distinct borders, Type III: ulcerative with indistinct borders, Type IV: diffuse, indistinct borders (see Japan Neoplastic Lesion classification below)

Carman-meniscus sign (on upper GI contrast study) – concavity (toward lumen) of large and flat gastric ulcers suggesting ulcerated malignancy as benign ulcers should be concave to the lumen. 'Meniscus sign' but itself could be representative of a concavity seen in a pleural effusion on chest x-ray

Isaacson-Wright disease AKA Gastric MALT lymphoma AKA MALToma AKA extranodal marginal zone B cell lymphoma – associated with H. pylori, chemo and radio-sensitive

Japan Neoplastic Lesion classification (Based on the older Borrman classification):

Type 0 - superficial polypoid, flat/depressed, or excavated tumours

Type 1 - polypoid carcinomas, usually attached on a wide base

Type 2 - ulcerated carcinomas with sharply demarcated and raised margins

Type 3 - ulcerated, infiltrating carcinomas without definite limits

Type 4 - nonulcerated, diffusely infiltrating carcinomas

Type 5 - unclassifiable advanced carcinomas

(see also the Paris classification in the colorectal section)

Krukenberg tumour – Matastasis to an ovary or ovaries typically from a pyloric gastric adenocarcinoma (though possible from other sources)

Lauren classification of Gastric Carcinoma – Intestinal (Differentiated, typically in older >50yr old patients, associated with H. pylori, metaplastic glands in chronic gastritis, male>female) vs. Diffuse (Undifferentitaed, e.g. linitis plastic and signet ring types, typically younger patients with no association with H. pylori, recently growing incidence)

Ménétrier's disease AKA Menetrier disease AKA hypoproteinemic hypertrophic gastropathy – Premalignant (for gastric cancer) comprising of giant gastric fold hyperplasia and excessive mucous production with no acid and protein loss. Are often hypochlorhydric (deficiency of stomach hydrochloric acid)

Siewert-Stein classification of oesophago-gastric junction tumours (adenocarcinoma) – Type I (distal part of the oesophagus, centre 1-5cm above OGJ), Type II (at the real cardia, within 1cm above and 2cm below the OGJ), Type III (subcardial stomach, 2-5cm below OGJ)

Signet Ring Cell – Large vacuole and mucin carrying, cancerous cell in several organs, most notable in stomach adenocarcinoma where it carries a poor prognosis

Gastric Resections

Billroth I AKA Pean-Billroth operation – Gastroduodenostomy (end-to-end). Modifications: Finney, Finsterer, Haberer I, Haberer II, Kocher, Rydygier, Shelton-Horsley, Shoemaker

Billroth II(a) operation – Gastrojejunostomy (side-to-side). Modification (end-to-side): Hofmeister (von Hofmeister), Finsterer (note: Finsterer-Hofmeister procedure is a partial gastrectomy with a retrocolic gastrojejunostomy at the greater curvature), Krönlein, Mikulicz, Polya (retrocolic end-to-side gastrojejunostomy), Reichel, von Eiselsberg, von Hacker

Billroth II(b) Braun Modification – Gastrojejunostomy (side-to-side) with Braun jejunojejunostomy

Billroth II(c) – Gastrojejunostomy (side-to-side) with Roux-en-Y construction. Modification: Moynihan, Whipple

Proximal Gastrectomy Types:

Oesophago-gastrostomy with: Direct oesophago-gastrostomy, gastric tube anastomosis, lower oesophageal sphincter preservation, fundoplication

Oesophago-jejunostomy by: Jejunal interposition (JI), Jejunal Pouch interposition (JPI), Double Tract reconstruction (DT)

12. GASTRIC (BENIGN) AND GASTRO-OESOPHAGEAL REFLUX

Anti-reflux Procedures

Belsey partial fundoplication AKA Belsey Mark IV Repair – 270° anterior transthoracic

Collis I procedure (Hiatoplasty) – Downward position of Gastro-oesophageal junction at the hiatus to restore the Angle of HIS

Collis II procedure AKA Collis gastroplasty – when wanting to perform a fundoplication with short oesophagus, vertical incision at left gastric border creates a longer pseudo-oesophageal conduit that offers length for the fundoplication. Typically performed with Nissen or Belsey Mark IV fundoplications

Dor partial Fundoplication– anterior 180–200°

Endoscopic Anti-reflux procedures– Esophyx, LINX

Guarner partial Fundoplication– 240° posterior

Hill Posterior Gastropexy – NOT FUNDOPLICATION, Hiatoplasty and gastropexy to right crura

Lind procedure – 300° posterior wrap fixation of the posterior wrap to the lateral oesophageal wall

Lortat-Jacob procedure – Cardiophrenopexy, reconstitutes 'standard' upper GI anatomy by freeing distal oesophagus, attaching the gastric fundus to the sub-diaphragmatic peritoneum, Angle of His reconstruction and oesophageal fixation to the right gastric fundus (based on technical experience with pelvic floor/ perineal weakness/prolapse)

Merendino Procedure I (Hiatotomy + Hiatoplasty)– (a)Thoracic Hiatoplasty/Phrenoplasty (diaphragmic hiatus incision) and repositioning of lower oesophagus through neo-hiatus (b)same procedure through abdomen approach

Merendino Procedure II – Jejunal cardioplasty (pedicled jejunal patch to form Gastric Cardia neo-sphinctre)

Nissen total fundoplication – 360°, intraoperative demonstration of the 'shoe-shine' manoeuvre demonstrating fundus free posteriorly prior to suturing the wrap

Nissen-Rossetti procedure – Nissen procedure without dividing/'taking down' the short gastric vessels

Toupet partial Fundoplication– 270° posterior ('Touposterior')

Thal partial Fundoplication – 270° anterior ('Thanterior')
Watson Procedure – 120° anterior, freeing distal

oesophagus, Angle of His reconstruction and oesophageal fixation to the crura

Berti-Berg Disease AKA Gastric Volvulus

Borchardt's Triad of Gastric Volvulus – acute epigastric pain, violent wretching, inability to pass NG tube. Three types of gastric volvulus AKA Berti-Berg Disease: (1) organoaxial axis linking the GOJ to the pylorus, (2) mesenteroaxial axis linking the lesser and greater curvatures, (3) mixed

Gastro-Oesophageal Reflux Disease

Congo red test – older test, invasive qualitative for measuring gastric acid secretion

DeMeester score AKA Johnston-DeMeester score – scores lower oesophageal acidity and proxy of GORD severity. It is based on six parameters (1) total reflux, (2) upright reflux, (3) supine reflux, (4) number of episodes, (5) number of episodes >5min, (6) longest episode

Heidelberg capsule – non-invasive quantitative test for measuring gastric acid secretion

Hiatus Hernia Types – part of stomach or intestine protrudes into chest due to diaphragmatic hiatus defect. Types: (1) Sliding upto 90%, Oesophago-gastric junction above diaphragm (2) Rolling (Para-oesophageal) (3) Mixed (4) Stomach/Bowel in chest

Horvath Classification – True vs Apparent Oesophageal Shortening

Los Angeles Endoscopic classification of the severity of reflux oesophagitis – A → D

Merendino Classification of Hiatus Hernia: (1) Short oesophagus with stomach in thorax (rare) (2) Stomach herniation through hiatus WITHOUT displacing oesophagus (paraoesophageal), (3) Stomach herniation through hiatus WITH displacing oesophagus

Minaire's score reflux – >4 reflects severity of acid reflux

Montreal Classification – GORD is a condition which develops when the reflux of stomach contents causes troublesome symptoms and/or complications.

(1)Oesophageal Syndromes: (a) Symptomatic (e.g. reflux, chest pain), (b) Symptomatic + Oesophageal Injury (e.g. oesophagitis, Barrett;'s)

(2)Extra-Oesophageal Syndromes: (a) Established Association (e.g. cough/ Asthma, laryngitis), (b) Proposed association (e.g. pharygitis or sinusitis)

Visick Classification of Upper GI Symptoms – (I) Asymptomatic, (II) Mild, (III) Moderate, (IV) Life incapacitating, (V) Worse than Preoperative

Gastric Ulcer Procedures:

Johnson classification of Gastric Ulcers – Type I-Lesser curvature near incisura, Type II (double)-Body and duodenum, Type III-prepyloric antrum, Type IV-cardia near GOJ, Type V-NSAIDS (anywhere). II and III result from acid hypersecretion and I, IV and V result from muscoal defence damage

Csendes procedure – Roux-en-Y gastro-jejunostomy for high ucers (Type IV near gastro-esophageal junction)

Kelling-Madlener Procedure – anterectomy and oversewing of ulcer

Pauchet Procedure – Billroth I type operation with antrectomy/ distal gastrectomy and extension of resection to excise ulcer along lesser curvature of stomach

Peptic Ulcer Disease

Armour operation – Lesser curvature gastroplasty: flap exteriorization of ulcer and formation of a gastric pouch

Graham patch AKA Graham Omentopexy – omental closure of peptic duodenal perforation. Note, in duodenal ulcers (without perforation) there is symptomatic relief with food consumption (temporary for 2-3 hours) and in gastric ulcers the pain is precipitated by food

Heineke-Mikulicz pyloroplasty (with truncal vagotomy) – longitudinal incision and transverse closure, not applicable in pyloric stenosis/ pyloric scarring

Finney pyloroplasty – side-to-side gastroduodenostomy with pyloromyotomy

Jaboulay pyloroplasty – side-to-side gastroduodenostomy without pyloromyotomy

Mayo operation – Transgastric Excision of ulcer of the posterior wall of the stomach

U-stich – suture ligation of gastroduodenal branches for bleeding peptic ulcer

13.   GASTRO-INTESTINAL DISEASES

Abdominal Angina – (1) postprandial pain, (2) 'fear to eat' weight loss (3) aortic/ abdominal bruit

Aretaeus' Cœliac Affection AKA Coeliac disease – autoimmune condition of the small bowel causing malabsorption, diarrhoea and bloating with abdominal distension (note Iron deficiency anaemia and B12/folate deficiency). Typically associated with other autoimmune conditions such as Type I Diabetes Mellitus, Autoimmune Thyroiditis etc. Several diagnostic tests including those for anti-endomysial (EMA) antibodies and anti-gliadin (AGA) antibodies. Associated with small bowel adenocarcinoma and Non-Hodgkins Lymphoma (T-cell lymphoma, NOT B-cell lymphoma)

Bassen-Kornzweig   syndrome   AKA Abetalipoproteinaemia – Autosomal recessive condition of fat absorption due to a microsomal triglyceride transfer protein mutation.

Broad   Beta   disease AKA   Familial Dysbetalipoproteinaemia   AKA   Type   III hyperlipoproteinaemia AKA Remnant hyperlipidaemia – Hereditary dyslipidaemia with deceased HDL

Chagas disease AKA Chagas' disease AKA American trypanosomiasis –Parasitic infection with the 'kissing-bug' protozoan Trypanosoma cruzi. Can cause Mega-oesophagus ('Sigmoid Oesophagus' – see below) and Megacolon

Curling's ulcer AKA Stress Ulcer – Gastric ulcers and erosions associated with severe burns/ trauma/ injury/ illness

Cushing ulcer AKA on Rokitansky-Cushing syndrome – gastric ulcer (or ulcer in the distal oesophagus or proximal duodenum) associated with raised intracranial pressure

Dieulafoy's lesion AKA Exulceratio Simplex Dieulafoy AKA Caliber-persistent artery AKA Gastric vessel aneurysm – tortuous submucosal arteriole(s), 75% of which exit within 6cm of the Gastro-oesophageal junction that can be a cause of upper gastro-intestinal bleeding

Grönblad–Strandberg syndrome AKA Pseudoxanthoma elasticum (PXE) – genetic connective tissue disorder (elastic fibres) causing GI bleeds and affects skin, eyes and blood, autosomal recessive

Heberden-Gee syndrome AKA abdominal migraine AKA cyclic vomiting syndrome (adult or child) – cyclical/recurrent abdominal pain with vomiting and generalised symptoms e.g. headache and crying. Treated with anti-emetic and anti-migraine medications

Lykoudis protocol – antibiotic management for peptic ulcer disease

Osler–Weber–Rendu disease AKA Osler–Weber–Rendu syndrome AKA Hereditary haemorrhagic telangiectasia (HHT) – GI bleeding, epistaxis, fragile punctiform blood vessels on mucous membranes. Autosomal dominant

Plumbi dolor AKA lead colic – abdominal pain from lead poisoning

Whipple's disease – systemic bacterial infection due to Tropheryma whipplei (Different Whipple to Whipple's operation). Typically presents with (1) diarrhoea) and (2) arthritis. Can have sub-total villous atrophy on histology, so is a differential for Coeliac disease, Norwalk virus/Norovirus and Tropical Sprue

Vampire/ Werewolf disease AKA Hoppe-Seyler disease AKA Stokvis disease AKA Schultz disease AKA Porphyria – condition of porphyrin build-up with multiple systemic effects, including those of abdominal pain, skin and neurological signs

Gastro-intestinal Haemorrhage:

Forrest classification – predictive classification of upper gastrointestinal haemorrhage. I-haemorrhage, II-recent haemorrhage, III- lesion without active bleeding

Glasgow-Blatchford – risk stratification tool to assess need for medical intervention in upper gastrointestinal bleeding

Linton–Nachlas tube – balloon inflatable tube for controlling oesophageal varices haemorrhage (no oesophageal component)

Minnesota tubes – modification of the Sengstaken–Blakemore tube with an opening at the proximal oesophageal end

Rockall score – used to stratify risk for upper gastrointestinal bleeding

Sengstaken–Blakemore – balloon inflatable tube for controlling oesophageal varices haemorrhage. Has an inferior gastric end opening

14. HAEMATOLOGY

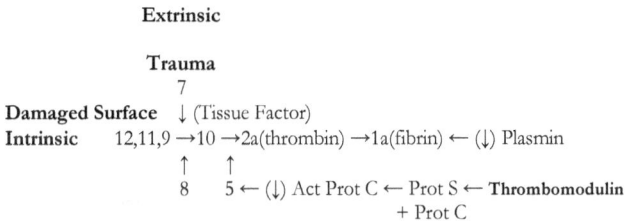

Extrinsic

Trauma
                7
Damaged Surface   ↓ (Tissue Factor)
Intrinsic   12,11,9 →10 →2a(thrombin) →1a(fibrin) ← (↓) Plasmin
                ↑   ↑
                8   5 ← (↓) Act Prot C ← Prot S ← **Thrombomodulin**
                                    + Prot C

Factor 12 (Hageman factor)
Prekallikrein (Fletcher factor)

Vitamin K dependent- 2, 7, 9, 10

PT – measures extrinsic system: 1, 2, 5, 7, 10
APTT – meaures instrinsic system: 1, 2, 5, 8, 9, 10, 11, 12

Auer bodies AKA Auer rods – Red staining, cytoplasmic structures, shaped as needlesin myeloblasts, or progranulocytes in some leukemias

Addison's anaemia AKA Biermer's anemia AKA Addison–Biermer anemia AKA Combe-Addison disease AKA pernicious anaemia AKA Vitamin B12 deficiency anaemia – presents with anaemia, and a triad of Paraesthesia, Glossitis (with red atrophic tongue) fatigue and general symptoms including 'the sighs' as shortness of breath. There is positivity for serum anti-intrinsic factor antibody

Burkitt lymphoma – B-cells in the germinal centre, c-myc gene proto-oncogene, associated with Epstein-Barr virus infection

Christmas disease AKA Haemophilia B – Factor IX deficiency

Classic Haemophilia AKA Haemophilia A – Factor VIII deficiency

Coombs test AKA Coombs' test AKA antiglobulin test (AGT) – test for auto-antibodies against red cells. Two types: (1) Direct, test for IgG alloantibodies (reacting with antigens from a genetically different individual of the same species), IgG autoantibodies and Complement proteins bound to the surface of red blood cells using anti-human globulin (also known as "Coombs reagent"). (2) Indirect, used prior to blood transfusion (in someone who's had a recent transfusion) or in pregnancy, testing for anti-RBC antibodies in serum

Fanconi anaemia – genetic disorder with (1) cancer (typically AML), (2) Bone marrow failure (3) congenital anomalies, (4) endocrinopathy and (5) developmental disabilities

Helmet Cells AKA schistocyte AKA schizocyte – fragmented red cells seen in microangiopathic diseasessuch as DIC (disseminated intravascular coagulation), severe aortic stenosis and mechanical heart valves

Hughes syndrome AKA Hughes-Harris-Gharavi Syndrome AKA Antiphospholipid syndrome AKA Antiphospholipid antibody syndrome. Hypercoagulable state due to antiphospholipid antibodies generating arterial and venous thrombi and other pregnancy-related issues (preterm delivery, preeclampsia, miscarriage and stillbirth). Can be primary or secondary (e.g. due to SLE). When severe can cause multiple organ failure and is known as Asherson syndrome or catastrophic antiphospholipid syndrome (CAPS)

ISTH (International Society on Thrombosis and Haemostasis) DIC Score: (>5 Overt DIC) –

Decreasing Platelet count: >100=0, 50-100=1, <50=2
Increased FDPs: none=0, moderate=2, strong=3
Increased PT: <3 sec=0, 3-6 sec=1, >6 sec=2
Decreased Fibrinogen: >100 mg/dl=0, <100 mg/dl=1

Factor V Leiden mutation AKA resistance to activated protein C – is a thrombotic clotting disorder where a mutated Factor V that normally functions as a cofactor for activated factor X but cannot be broken down by activated protein C (which typically degrades it) resulting in thrombosis. Skin necrosis is a noted complication in these patients when they are on warfarin therapy

Transfusion haemolytic reaction groups – ABO, Rhesus, Kell, Duffy, Kidd, ALSO P and MN systems (though rarely)

Non-haemolytic reaction groups – Lutheran, Lewis, Scianna, Li

Negus technique AKA St. Thomas's Hospital technique – isotope labelled (125I) fibrinogen uptake method of detecting DVT

Owren's disease – Factor V deficiency

Purpura Fulminans – acute life threatening pro-thrombotic clotting disorder seen typically as a result of Protein C deficiency or deficiency of its co-factor (Protein S). Both are vitamin K dependent. Together they degrade Factor Va and VIIIa.

Reed–Sternberg cells AKA lacunar histiocytes – 'owl's eye' appearance, noted in Hodgkin's lymphoma (typically CD30 and CD15 positive and CD20 and CD45 negative). Can also be seen in infectious mononucleosis and carbamazepine lymphadenopathy. Hodgkin lymphoma more common as a cause of mediastinal lymphadenopathy <10yrs (Reed-Sternberg) and Non-Hodgkin 10-30yrs (B, T cell clonality). Both can present with coughing, dyspnoea, dysphagia and haemoptysis. They can also demonstrate 'B symptoms' : fever, night sweating and weight loss (typically in more aggressive disease)

Splenectomy cells:

Howell Jolly Bodies
Heinz Bodies
Target Cells AKA Mexican Hat Cells AKA Bullseye cells AKA Codocytes AKA Leptocytes AKA Poikilocytosis
Siderocyte (red cells containing non-haeme iron)
Pappenheimer bodies (tested with May-Grünwald Giemsa and Perls' Prussian blue stain)

Stuart–Prower factor AKA Factor X

Vaquez disease AKA Osler-Vaquez disease AKA

Polycythemia rubra vera – Bone marrow neoplasm producing excess red blood cells

von Willebrand disease – is an autosomal dominant bleeding disorder due to missing or defective von Willebrand factor; a protein that (1) binds and potentiates factor VIII and (2) also supports platelets function. It is treated by Desmopressin, sold under the trade name DDAVP (also used for diabetes insipidus and Haemophilia A) which releases von Willebrand Factr from the Weibel-Palade bodies of endothelial cells

Waldenström macroglobulinaemia (WM) – rare type of non-Hodgkin lymphoma

Warfarin/ Coumadin reversal – in emergency use Prothrombin complex concentrate (PCC) AKA Factor IX complex – factors II, IX, X (occasionally VIII), Trade names: Beriplex, Octaplex, Kcentra, others

Werlhof's disease AKA ITP AKA Immune thrombocytopaenic purpura – typically acute in children and chronic in adults

15. HEPATOBILIARY

AAST (American Association of the Surgery of Trauma) classification of pancreatic injury – I-minor contusion without duct injury, II-major contusion without duct injury, III-distal + ductal injury, IV-proximal (right of SMV) + ductal injury, V-massive head disruption

Alagille syndrome – Genetic condition typically affecting the liver and heart (but also other organs). Can present with jaundice and biliary atresia with congenital cardiac disease.

Alsono-Lej classification – choledochal cysts

Bismuth–Corlette Classification (of peri-hilar cholangiocarcinomas) – identifies location and longitudinal extension of biliary tree tumours. Types I-IV (see also Stewart-Way, Hannover and Strasberg classifications)

Belghiti 50-50 Criteria AKA Belghiti score – Predicitive score of liver failure and mortality after hepatectomy. It consists of prothrombin index and bilirubin, with threshold values based on the Child-Pugh score

Bouveret syndrome – Gastric outlet obstruction and proximal gallstone ileus secondary to gallstone in the proximal duodenum or pylorus

Budd-Chiari – occlusion of the hepatic veins with 1.Pain, 2. Ascites, 3.Liver Failure (Acute Fulminant or Chronic)

Calot Triangle AKA Calot's Triangle AKA Cystohepatic Triangle – potential space at porta hepatis where the cystic artery and cystic duct can be found. (Right) Cystic Duct, (Left) Common Hepatic Duct, (Superior) Inferior surface of the liver

Calot's node AKA Node of Lund – lymph node in Calot's triangle

Cantlie's line – conceptual line dividing the liver into left and right lobes in hepatectomy procedures, it extends from the inferior vena cava to the middle of the gallbladder fossa

Charcot's cholangitis triad – jaundice; fever (typically with rigors) right upper quadrant (RUQ) abdominal pain

Child-Pugh Score for Cirrhosis Mortality AKA Child–Turcotte–Pugh score – consists of (1) bilirubin, (2) albumin, (3) PT, (4) encephalopathy, (5) ascites. Ranges from 5-15, >7 can be considered for transplantation

Couinaud classification – Classification of hepatic segments I-VIII

Courvoisier's law AKA Courvoisier syndrome AKA Courvoisier's sign AKA Courvoisier-Terrier's sign – Painless jaundice associated with a non-tender palpably enlarged gallbladder is unlikely to be gallstones, and possibly an upper GI malignancy (e.g. pancreatic). This is because inflamed gallbladders typically become fibrotic and shrink

Disse (Space of) – perisinusoidal space

Double barrel sign – ultrasound finding of biliary dilatation, usually >7mm

Double duct sign – concomitant dilatation of the CBD and pancreatic ducts. Typically seen in ampullary (Ampulla of Vater) or pancreatic head cancers

Duncan Cholecystitis AKA Acalculous Cholecystitis – non-stone gallbladder inflammation seen in severe illness(sepsis, burns etc), trauma, vasculitis, mesenteric atherosclerosis, or infections e.g typhoid or Salmonella

Edmondson disease – Focal nodular hyperplasia, associated with stellate central scar in 60-70%, also associated with oral contraceptive use

Erythromycin obstructivus – obstructive jaundice picture (extra-hepatic) of erythromycin

Fish mouth ampulla – Main duct IPMN (seen in 1/3 of main duct IPMN)

Gilbert's syndrome – mild jaundice due to increased unconjugated bilirubin (several different genotypic variants)

Glissonian AKA Glissonean approach – utilisation of the Glisson's capsule, the hilar plate and the Glissonian/ Glissonean pedicles for liver resection surgery

Goppert-Kalckar disease AKA Galactosaemia – Genetic diseae of metabolism with symptoms of jaundice, diarrhoea and vomiting. Can lead to severe neurological disease

Hannover Classification of Bile Duct Injuries – identifies location and longitudinal extension of biliary tree tumours. Type A-E (see also Bismuth-Corlette, Stewart-Way and Strasberg classifications)

Heaney manoeuvre – total vascular isolation of the liver by clamping the inferior vena cava, below and above below the liver, can be performed in conjunction with Pringle's manoevre

Kasai procedure – Roux-en Y hepato-porto-enterostomy for biliary atresia

Klatskin tumor AKA hilar cholangiocarcinoma – cholangiocarcinoma at the convergence point of the right and left hepatic bile ducts

Kayser-Fleischer rings – copper deposits in the corneal membrane associated with Wilson's disease

Kocherisation of the duodenum AKA Kocher's manoeuvre – dissection (lateral) of the duodenum (+/- pancreas head) off the retroperitoneum. Can be extended by a Kocher+ manoeuvre AKA Cattell-Brasch manoeuvre toward the right white line of Toldt and subsequently across the small bowel mesenteric root. This begins at begins at the common bile duct and ends at the ligament of Treitz. This exposes the inframesocolic retroperitoneum, IVC, infra-renal aorta, both renal hila, both iliac vessels and superior mesenteric vessels (can be used in Trauma and Vascular Surgery)

Kocher incision – right subcostal incision (see also Kocher incision in thyroid/endocrine surgery)

Kuppfer cells AKA Stellate macrophages AKA Kupffer-Browicz cells AKA 'Sternzellen' – cells in contact with hepatocytes (in association with reticuloendothelial cells) that are involved in synthesising unconjugated bilirubin in the liver from biliverdin (in turn from haemoglobin and myoglobin). As toxic this is bound to albumin in the circulation. Conjugation by heptocytes are typically with glucuronic acid

LABEL procedure – Laser-Assisted Bile Duct Exploration by Laparoendoscopy for Choledocholithiasis

Laurell-Eriksson disease AKA Alpha1-Antitrypsin Deficiency AKA A1AD – Inherited disease typically affecting (1) Lungs (emphysema, COPD), (2) Liver (cirrhosis, autoimmune hepatitis), (3) Blood

Lortat-Jacob procedure AKA controlled right hepatectomy – anatomical right hepatectomy with hepatoduodenal ligament dissection of the hepatic artery, portal vein and bile duct

Lower-Farrell syndrome – splenic artery aneurysm bleeding through the pancreatic duct, see also Vankemmel wirsungorrhagia

Luschka's duct – Accessory bile duct from the liver, biliary tree or right hepatic ductal system into the gallbladder

MELD AKA Model for End-Stage Liver Disease – score for assessing chronic liver disease (see Child–Pugh score)

Mercedes incision – Tripartite incision to gain access to the liver and pancreas

Mirizzi's syndrome – compression of the common bile

duct (CBD) or common hepatic duct (typically causing jaundice) as a result of an impacted gallstone at the cystic duct or neck of the gallbladder. Classified by McSherry as: Type I direct compression and/or local inflammation of the CBD, Type II Mirizzi's syndrome, stone erosion into the CBD with fistulation. Subsequently classified by Csendes adding: Type III fistula 2/3 circumference of CBD, Type IV fistula comprises the whole circumference of CBD, Type V corresponds to any type of Mirizzi associated with a bilioenteric fistula with or without gallstone ileus

Murphy sign – pain exacerbation on sub-costal, mid-clavicular pressure on inspiration

Paget's disease AKA osteitis deformans – bone disorder with raised alkaline phosphatase due to severe bone breakdown and disorganised reformation/ remodelling

Pringle manoeuvre AKA Anterior Winslow Foramen manoeuvre– pressure/ clamping of the hepato-duodenal ligament to minimise bleeding during surgery. It is located at the free border of the lesser omentum containing the portal triad, laterally to medial: (1) CBD, (2) Portal vein and (3) Common hepatic artery

Reye's (Ryes) syndrome – Encephalopathy and liver failure associated with concomitant viral infection and aspirin use (typically in children though a few adult cases have been noted)

Reynolds cholangitis pentad –Charcot's triad + shock and an altered mental status.

Rigler's Triad of Gallstone Ileus – (1) small bowel obstruction, (2) aerobilia, (3) gallstone outside gallbladder

Rokitansky–Aschoff sinuses – pseudodiverticula of the gallbladder associated with adenomyomatosis (benign). On CT: 'teething ring' and also the 'rosary sign'. On MRI: 'pearl necklace sign'

Saint's triad – (1) Gallstones (cholelithiasis), (2) Hiatus hernia, (3) Diverticular disease

Spider Naevi AKA Spider Angioma AKA Nevus Araneus AKA vascular spider AKA spider telangiectasia – telangiectasia associated with liver disease

Stewart-Way Classification of Bile Duct Injuries – identifies location and longitudinal extension of biliary tree tumours. Classes I-IV (see also Bismuth-Corlette, Hannover and Strasberg classifications)

Stoltz Disease AKA May-Strong Disease – Emphysematous Cholecystitis

Strasberg Classification of Bile Duct Injuries – Classes A-E (see also Bismuth-Corlette, Hannover and Stewart-Way classifications)

Sunburst central calcification – seen in Pancreatic Serous Cystadenoma, typically with honeycomb morphology

Sump Syndrome – Repeat acute cholangitis at hepatico-jejunostomy (possibly due to bacterial overgrowth or altered bile circultion)

Todani Classification (modification of the Alsono-Lej classification) – choledochal cysts:
(1)Extrahepatic bile duct, (a)entire, (b)segment, (c) CBD
(2)CBD diverticulum
(3)Choledochocele, cyst in duodenum

(4)Intra- + Extra-haptic ducts (multiple)
(5) Intra-hepatic duct dilatations. Caroli disease, associated with benign renal tubular ectasia. Represents other spectrum end of fibropolycystic disease AKA Von Meyenburg complexes AKA biliary hamartomas
[(6)] Newer (not classical Todani), Cystic Duct

Tokyo classification AKA Tokyo Guidelines for the management of acute cholangitis and cholecystitis

Trousseau disease AKA Haemochromatosis type 1 AKA hereditary haemochromatosis AKA HFE gene-related hereditary haemochromatosis – (1) excess dietary absorption of iron, (2) excess iron body stores. Results in with cirrhosis, polyarthropathy, adrenal insufficiency, heart failure, diabetes, slatey-grey skin pigmentation, testicular atrophy, impotence. Noted particularly in Celtic descent individuals

Tsuchida anti-reflux valve AKA Nakajo-Tsuchida anti-reflux valve – An intussusception-type antireflux valve for the Roux-en-Y loop after a Kasai operation in patients with biliary atresia to prevent episodes of ascending cholangitis

Tung-Quang Procedure – Right hepatectomy with ligation of ligated the portal pedicles intra-hepatically after liver parenchyma dissection

Vankemmel Wirsungorrhagia AKA Hemosuccus pancreaticus AKA Pseudohematobilia – bleeding in pancreatic duct from peri-pancreatic structures such as the splenic artery, see Lower-Farrell Syndrome

Wagner Disease AKA Peliosis Hepatis – benign condition with dilatation of sinusoidal and perisinusoidal (Disse space; see above) areas

Wilson's disease – Rare autosomal recessive condition (mutation in ATP7B gene) causing (1) Neurological and (2) Liver originating symptoms. Patients may present with Kayser-Fleischer rings in the eye, low serum caeruloplasmin and low blood copper levels. High urinary copper levels and amino-aciduria. They can also present with Parkinsoniansim

16.   HERNIAS

Hernias, Femoral

Cooper (to scrotum or labia via femoral canal)
Cloquet AKA Callison-Cloquet (pectineal)
Femoral canal
Hesselbach (external femoral) lateral to femoral vessels under the inguinal ligament
De Laugier AKA Laugier (lacunar ligament)
Narath or Teale (prevascular), behind femoral artery seen in congenital dislocation of the hip
Serafini (retrovascular)
Velpeau (prevascular)

Repair

McEvedy (High or Suprainguinal) – Originally Vertical/ Paramedian (later modified to transverse), conjoint to Cooper's ligament (AKA Pectineal ligament). Retroperitoneal. **Nyhus incision** AKA Nyhus-Cheattle-McEvedy retroperitoneal approach. Modified McEvedy half-Pfannenstiel incision

Lotheissen (Inguinal) – Transversalis approach, sac resected, conjoint tendon is sutured to Cooper's ligament (iliopectineal ligament)

Lockwood (Low) – Sac resected and inguinal ligament sutured to Cooper's ligament (Pectineal)

Kugel Mesh Retroperitoneal Repair – using Rives and Stoppa wide mesh cover technique

Hernias, Inguinal

Gilmore's Groin AKA Athletic pubalgia AKA Sports hernia AKA Hockey hernia/ groin – groin pain over the pubic tubercle typically seen in athletes and typically associated with a dilated external inguinal ring

Poupart's ligament = Inguinal ligament (4cm from ASIS to pubic tubercle)

Poupart's canal: Oblique except in newborns

Floor – Poupart's/ Inguinal ligament + Gimbernat/ Lacunar ligament
Roof – Internal oblique and Transversus abdominis
Posterior – Fascia transversalis and Conjoint tendon
Anterior – Aponeurosis of the external oblique muscle and internal oblique muscle in its lateral third

Differential in women:

Nuck Hydrocoele AKA Hydrocoele of the canal of Nuck – Failure of obliteration/ Persistence of the processus vaginalis peritonei in females

Silk-glove sign – texture of indirect sac on paediatric hernias

Zieman – Three Finger Test

Anatomy

Bogros' space AKA retro-inguinal space – sub-inguinal ligament sandwiched between the transversalis fascia transversalis anteriorly and the peritoneum posteriorly. The iliac fascia lies laterally. Communicates with the space of Retzius

Cloquet's node AKA Rosenmüller's node – most superior of deep inguinal lymph nodes or most inferior of external iliac lymph nodes (please note Cloquet's canal in ophthalmology)

Cooper's Ligament = Pectineal ligament = Iliopectineal ligament

Gimbernat's Ligament = Lacunar ligament (medial to femoral canal)

Hesselbach's triangle AKA inguinal triangle – Triangle through which direct hernia's come through. Base (inguinal or Poupart's ligament), Medial (lateral border of the rectus sheath), Lateral (inferior epigastric vessels)

Retzius space AKA cave of Retzius – retropubic space (also Striae of Retzius on enamel). Communicates with the space of Borgos

Hernia Types

Amyand – (indirect) containing appendix in inguial hernia (Note Losanoff-Basson and Athena classifications)

De Garengeot – containing appendix in femoral hernia

Hernia-en-glissade AKA Sliding– retroperitoneal viscus as part of sac

Littre's – (indirect) containing Meckel's diverticulum

Maydl's AKA Hernia-en-W – W-shaped

Romberg AKA Pantaloon AKA Saddle AKA dual – concurrent direct and indirect hernias

Richter's – hernia incorporating part of small bowel wall

Hernia Treatments:

Herniorraphy (Herniotomy [excision of sac] + posterior wall strengthening)

Bassini (Conjoint sutured to inguinal)
McVey (Transversus abdominis aponeurosis to Cooper's ligament (pectineal) and iliopubic tract)
Shouldice (Conjoint sutured to inguinal, Double breast Transversalis, Transversus abdominis aponeurosis to iliopubic tract)

Hernioplasty (Herniorraphy + prosthesis)

Lichtenstein Mesh Repair

TEP balloon plane – Between rectus muscle and

posterior rectus sheath

Hernia's, Obturator

de Ronsil Hernia AKA Ronsil Hernia AKA de Ronsil-Obre Hernia – Obturator Hernia

Howship-Romberg Sign: medial thigh and hip pain with external rotation and extension

Hannington-Kiff Sign: absent thigh adductor reflex with a positive patellar reflex (secondary to compression of the obturator nerve)

Hernia's, Other

Garré benign intestinal stenosis AKA Garré-Guignard stenosis – small bowel stenosis following successful reduction of a strangulated hernia

Grynfeltt-Lesshaft Hernia AKA Grynfeltt-Lesshaft-Petit Hernia – Lumbar Hernia

Incisional – Can be repaired by the Rives-Stoppa retromuscular, preperitoneal sublay method

Mayo Repair AKA 'vest over pants' repair – for umbilical and paraumbilical hernias

Ogilvie AKA Basuga (Area in Africa) AKA Funicular Direct Inguinal Hernia – conjoint tendon

Spigelian – between rectus abdominis muscle medially, and the semilunar line laterally

Parastomal – around a stoma, can be repaired by the (1) Sugarbaker technique or (2) Sandwich technique

Ramirez technique AKA component separation technique

TAR – Transversus abdominis release

17. LEGAL AND ETHICAL

Beauchamp-Childress four prima facie principles – (i)autonomy, (ii)beneficence, (iii)non-maleficence, (iv)justice

Bolam test AKA Bolamization – test to asses the 'duty of care' between a doctor and his/her patient, where the standard of that care is a matter of medical judgement. Used in Sidaway v. Board of Governors of the Bethlem Royal Hospital [1985] AC 871

Bolitho test – modification of the Bolam test, consists of two parts: (1) whether practitioner acted in accordance with accepted practice and (2) whether this was 'responsible' and 'logical'

Gillick competence – The capacity for an individual <16yrs to give or withhold consent to medical/surgical treatment/intervention

Montgomery ruling AKA Supreme Court's judgment in Montgomery v Lanarkshire Health Board – The doctor is therefore under a duty to take reasonable care to ensure that the patient is aware of any material risks involved in any recommended treatment, and of any reasonable alternative or variant treatments. The test of materiality is whether, in the circumstances of the particular case, a reasonable person in the patient's position would be likely to attach significance to the risk, or the doctor is or should reasonably be aware that the particular patient would be likely to attach significance to it. This is currently the standard in the UK

Consent Principles – **VICE**
Voluntary (no coercion)
Informed (Fully)
Capacity
Evidence (written, verbal or non-verbal/implied)

Summary: Bolam, consensus of reasonable body of practitioners (i.e doctors), Montgomery, reasonable body of patients, so patient-centric, no longer doctor-centric

18. MISCELLANEOUS

Abdominal Apoplexy – older term for (1) Mesenteric Vascular Infarction/ Thrombosis or (2) Intraperitoneal or retroperitoneal infarction/thrombosis

Alexander-Kotzareff procedure – Thoracic Sympathectomy

Alport syndrome – Genetic condition with (1) renal disease (glomerulonephritis, end-stage kidney disease and typically haematuria) (2) Hearing loss and (3) Occular abnormalities

'Anal wink' AKA Anal Reflex – S3,S4 nerves

Antibiotic Complications:

Red Man Syndrome (with Stevens-Johnson syndrome), Tinnitus and Ototoxicity – Vancomycin
Zooarthropathy – Ciprofloxacin (hence contraindicated in pregnancy/ children)
Ototoxicity and Nephrotoxicity – Gentamicin (gram negative cover)

Dens brunneis – Tetracycline brown teeth (hence contraindicated in pregnancy/ children)
Polyneuropathy, metallic taste and zoocarcinogenesis – Metronidazole (gram negative cover)

Bacon Lettuce and Tomato (BLT) with Kosher Pickles – Pneumonic for tumours metastasising to bone (typically lytic EXCEPT prostate): Breast, Lung, Thyroid, Kidney, Prostate

Baker's cyst –Excess knee joint fluid putting pressure on its posterior soft tissues

Battle's sign – post auricular bruising as a sign of basal skull fracture

Beaver muscle – Extensor carpi radialis brevis

Benediction hand – median nerve injury, typically seen when trying to make a fist (see Spinster's claw/ Ulnar Claw)

Berger's disease – IgA nephropathy responsible for the most common cause of glomerulonephritis globally, likely on the clinical spectrum of Henoch-Schönlein purpura

Berna classification – for rectus sheath haematomas based on CT findings: Type I (unilateral and contained within the muscle), Type II (either unilateral or bilateral and have blood between muscle and transversalis fascia), Type III (invading the prevesical space or peritoneum and may or may not affect the muscle)

Bible cyst AKA Bible bump AKA Gideon's disease AKA Olamide's cyst – Ganglion cyst (benign wrist tumour)

Bier block AKA Bier's block – Intravenous Regional

Anaesthesia

Biot's respiration – pathological breathing with rapid shallow inspirations followed by apnea episodes (regular or irregular)

Boari bladder flap – Ureteric reimplantation technique for long segment (>5cm) ureteric disease

Bouchard's nodes – proximal interphalangeal joint bony/ gelatinous cysts associated with osteoarthritis (see also Heberden's nodes)

Bovie diathermy – application of electrosurgical dissection and haemostasis. Can be monopolar or bipolar, and can incorporate (i) cutting, (ii) blended cut and coagulate, (iii) coagulate (pinpoint) low power AKA dessicate and (iv) coagulate high power (spray) AKA flugurate

Brain-Phalen Syndrome AKA Carpal Tunnel Syndrome – symptomatic condition of median nerve compression at the wrist

Burkitt's nasopharyngeal carcinoma – associated with Epstein-Barr virus, 7x more common in black than white children and can present with cervical lymphadenopathy (see also Burkitt lymphoma, B cells found in the germinal centre)

Celsus' Criteria for Inflammation – Rubor (Redness), Tumor (Swelling/Growth), Calor (Heat) and Dolor (Pain)

Cheyne-Stokes breathing – strenuous and faster breathing (crescendo-diminuendo) escalating to apneas and hyperpneoeas. Seen in chronic cardiac failure or respiratory centre damage

Chilaiditi syndrome AKA Chilaiditi sign of pseudo-pneumoperitoneum – anterior colonic position superior to the liver edge so that it directly abuts the under-surface of the right hemidiaphragm associated with right upper quadrant (RUQ) abdominal pain

Chlorosis AKA green sickness – Hypochromic anaemia

Clavien-Dindo AKA Clavien-Demartines-Dindo Classification – For surgical complications:

Grade I-Any deviation from the normal postoperative course without the need for pharmacological treatment or surgical, endoscopic and radiological interventions. Acceptable therapeutic regimens are: drugs as antiemetics, antipyretics, analgesics, diuretics and electrolytes and physiotherapy. This grade also includes wound infections opened at the bedside.
Grade II-Requiring pharmacological treatment with drugs other than such allowed for grade I complications. Blood transfusions and total parenteral nutrition are also included.
Grade III-Requiring surgical, endoscopic or radiological intervention, (a)intervention not under general anaesthesia, (b)intervention under general anaesthesia
Grade IV-Life-threatening complication (including CNS complications) requiring IC/ICU/ITU-management, (a)single organ dysfunction (including dialysis), (b)multi-organ dysfunction
Grade V-Death of a patient

Colles' fracture – common extra-articular fractures of the distal radius with doral (posterior) and radial displacement

Corneal arcus – hypercholesterolaemia and hyperlipoproteinaemia, lipid predominantly in two areas of the peripheral corneal stroma: (1) next to Bowman layer and (2) next to Descemet's membrane

CREST syndrome – Calcinosis, Raynaud's phenomenon, Esophageal dysmotility (with dysphagia), sclerodactyly, and telangiectasia, associated with systemic sclerosis and scleroderma. Upto 10% may suffer from primary biliary cirrhosis

De Quervain tenosynovitis AKA Texting thumb – thumb tenosynovitis

Dietl Syndrome AKA Wandering Spleen AKA Pelvic Spleen – weak or absent peri-splenic ligaments such that the spleen is not located at its usual position at the left upper quadrant splenic flexure

Double crush syndrome AKA Upton and McComas Syndrome – Carpal tunnel syndrome + peripheral nerve lesion (nerve compression/ irritation) higher-up (or lower-down) along the same nerve (e.g. C5/C6 nerve root) for Median nerve. An example for the Ulnar nerve is compression/ irritation at Guyon's tunnel and Cubital tunnel. For the Radial nerve there can be Radial Tunnel syndrome and a Cervical nerve root lesion.

Durand–Nicolas–Favre disease AKA Poradenitis inguinale AKA Strumous bubo AKA Climatic Bubo – Lymphogranuloma venereum that can cause inguinal lymphadenopathy

Dupuytren's Contracture – Thickening of palmar aponeurosis, particularly of ring and little finger, associated with diabetes, smoking, low BMI and Peyronie's disease BUT NO LONGER associated with the use of heavy vibrating machinery, alcohol, epilepsy, anti-epileptic drugs or liver disease

ERAS (Enhanced Recovery After Surgery) AKA **Kehlet Approach**

Erb's palsy AKA Erb–Duchenne palsy AKA Waiter's tip pasly – injury to the upper roots of the brachial plexus C5–C6 nerves

Ewing's sarcoma – paediatric bone tumour' usually in long bones (e.g. femur), is 30x more common in Caucasian children when compared to African or Afro-Caribbean children. Presents with pain, fever and occasionally pathological fractures

Falciform ligament sign AKA Silver sign – Pneumoperitoneum is present as intra-peritoneal gas surrounds and therefore exposes the falciform ligament. Usually present concurrently with Rigler's sign

Fitz-Hugh–Curtis syndrome – Peri-liver capsule adhesions in the context of pelvic inflammatory disease

Froment's sign – Test for ulnar nerve palsy due to weakness at adductor pollicis. When seen in conjunction with thumb metacarpophalangeal joint hyperextension it is known as Jeanne's Sign

Fowler's positions – Patient sitting with straight legs and hips flexed at Low (15-30 degrees), Semi (30-45 degrees), Standard (45-60 degrees), and High (80-90 degrees)

Garrod's nodes – subcutaneous proximal inter-phalangeal joint 'knuckle pads' composed of benign fibrofatty tissue

Ghon focus – lung lesion, subpleural typically mid to lower zone due to primary tuberculosis. Notable on x-rays (see also collar-stud abscess and Scrofula)

Gastrostomy Types – Janeway (elephant trunk), Stamm (circular suturing), Witzel (perpendicular straight sutures)

Halsted's principles AKA Tenets of Halsted – H: Haemostasis, A: Apposition of tissues, L: Lenient tissue handling, S: Sepsis minimisation, T: Tension minimisation, E: Ensuring vascular supply, D: Deadspace exclusion

Hasson penumoperitoneum technique AKA (mistakenly as the Hassan technique)

Heberden's nodes – distal interphalangeal joint bony/ gelatinous cysts associated with osteoarthritis (see also Bouchard's nodes)

Hoffa's fat pad – Infrapatellar fat pad
Hoffmann sign AKA Patel's sign AKA Trotter-Davies sign – percussion over a nerve demonstrates tingling sensation in a regenerated nerve (similar to Tinel's sign, related to Phalen's test)

Holmes-Adie pupil – tonically dilated pupil reacting slowly (to light) and a stronger accommodation reflex

Horner's syndrome – sympathetic trunk damage leading to (1) miosis, (2) ptosis , (3) apparent anhidrosis, (4) enophthalmos (in some cases)

Hounsfield unit (HU) – used in CT scanning where it is proportional to the degree of x-ray attenuation linked to each pixel to as an indicator of tissue density. Water has 0 HU and air has -1000 HU

Hudson mask – variable performance mask

Jackknife position AKA Kraske position – patient prone with hips flexed so that the hips are higher than both the head and legs

Jackson-Pratt drain – surgical drain with vacuum /suction device (used typically in neck or breast surgery), the 'Redivac' drain is a variant of this (see Penrose drain and Robinson drain)

Jenkin's Rule – suture length-to-wound length ratio for abdominal wounds is optimal at 4:1 or more (i.e. 6:1), less than this may lead to a 'burst abdomen'

Kimura's disease – Rare chronic inflammatory disorder presenting with painless head or neck lymphadenopathy

Klumpke's paralysis – lower root brachial plexus injury, C8, T1 (deep ulnar) nerve lesion causing claw hand

Koilonychia – Iron deficiency anaemia

Kussmaul respiration – strenuous inspirations associated with severe metabolic acidosis, noted in conditions such as diabetic ketoacidosis (DKA) and renal failure

Li-Fraumeni syndrome AKA SBLA syndrome – germline mutations of the p53 tumour suppressor gene resulting in cancers of sarcoma, breast, leukaemia and adrenal gland

Lindbergh operation – the first trans-atlantic operation performed by utilising a tele-robotic system (Zeus) where the robotic surgical device (and French surgeons) were in New York and the patient was in Strasbourg, France

Lesch–Nyhan syndrome AKA Nyhan syndrome AKA Juvenile gout – hypoxanthine-guanine phosphoribosyltransferase deficiency (HGPRT deficiency) presenting with (1) hyperuricosuric hyperuricemia (Gout and kidney disease) (2) Neurological disease and learning difficulties (3) vitamin B12 misabsorption and therefore megaloblastic anaemia. Presents between 3-6 months

Lloyd-Davies position – surgical position used in many colorectal and pelvic operations

Montandon tube – J-shaped tracheal tube

Maylard Transverse Muscle Cutting Incision – used for pelvic access, typically parallel (transverse) and approximately 2-5cm higher than the Pfannenstiel incision

Meigs' syndrome AKA Meigs syndrome AKA Demons-Meigs syndrome – Triad (1) Ascites, (2) Pleural effusion (3) Benign ovarian tumour (e.g. Brenner tumour [subtype of surface epithelial-stromal tumour], ovarian fibroma, fibrothecoma, granulosa cell tumour)

Meralgia paresthetica – Lateral cutaneous nerve of the thigh damage leading to lateral upper thigh numbness

Mittelschmerz – mid ovarian cycle pain

Munchausen syndrome – factitious psychiatric disorder of attention-seeking where patients fake symptoms and apply techniques to suggest organic evidence of their pseudo-illness

Munchausen syndrome by Proxy – Munchausen syndrome performed on an individual by someone else, for example a parent on a child (again in a self-attention seeking aim)

Nail signs – (see Koilonychia) Beau's lines (fingernail or toenail grooves associated with an episode of longstanding systemic disease), Mees' lines AKA Aldrich–Mees' lines AKA leukonychia striata (white discolouration signs)

associated with heavy metal poisoning (commonly Thallium), arsenic poisoning, chemotherapy and renal failure. Muehrcke's nails AKA Muehrcke's lines are similr to Mees' lines and also known as leukonychia striata or apparent leukonychia, and are white ail bed striata associated with nephrotic syndrome, hypoalbuminaemia and chemotherapy (see also thyroid nail disease). Parrot-beak nails AKA Kandil sign, this can be primary or secondary due to finger pulp atrophy as a result of conditions such as fingertip trauma, poor perfusion/ distal ischaemia after digit surgery and cocaine use. Plummer's nail, onycholysis (nail separation from the nail bed) typically in the ring and little fingers in thyrotoxicosis. Splinter haemorrhages (psoriasis, infective endocarditis, IV drug abuse, cardiac valve surgery, rheumatic heart disease, congenital cardiac disease, SLE and antiphospholipid syndrome). Red lunula (collagen diseases, systemic diseases, vascular diseases, cardiac failure, carbon monoxide poisoning and COPD). Yellow nail syndrome seen in systemic diseases and lymphoedema

Notta's nodule – nodule in metacarpophalangeal joint region associated with trigger fingers and stenosing tenosynovitis and a flexor tendon nodule of the Anterior pulley system. Typically seen congenitally in children's thumbs, though also presents on other digits throughout adulthood associated with inflammatory hand conditions

Oberg-Manske-Tonkin (OMT) Classification – For congenital anomalies of the hand and upper limb

Parona's space – space between pronator quadratus and the flexor tendons of the forearm

Phalen's test AKA Phalen's manoeuvre – test for carpal tunnel syndrome, performed by forced flexion at the wrist resulting in nerve compression in the carpal tunnel to generate its characteristics symptoms of tingling, numbness and burning. Can also be produced by the 'Reverse-Phalen's' where the wrist if forcibly extended

Pigbel AKA Pig Bel AKA Enteritis necroticans – Segmental necrotizing infection of the jejunum and ileum secondary to Clostridium perfringens Type C

PCPC GOV – Brain stem death, when unconscious (GCS=3), Pupils (fixed non-reacting), Corneal reflex (absent), Pain (no response), Cough (none, no tracheal reflex), Gag (none, no pharyngeal reflex), Occulo-vestibular reflex (none), Ventilatory effort (none, when mechanical ventilation is withdrawn for 5 minutes (with O2 at 5l/min via endotracheal cannula; PaCO2 >6.0 KPa and pH <7.4)

Penrose drain – soft surgical drain that collapses unless the pressure of fluid keeps it open (see Jackson-Pratt drain and Robinson drain)

Pfannenstiel incision – transverse skin fold incision approximately 5 cm above symphysis pubis used typically in obstetrics and gynaecology, pelvic surgery and modified in the modern McEvedy procedure for femoral hernia repair

Popeye sign – Rupture of the long head of the biceps tendon, resembling the upper arm muscle shape of the cartoon character Popeye

Prehn's sign – used to differentiate epididymitis and testicular torsion. In cases of painful testicles, if the pain is relieved due to elevation of the affected testicle, this is likely due to epididymitis rather than torsion (surgical emergency).

Raccoon eyes – peri-orbital bruising as a sign of basal skull fracture

Reye syndrome AKA Reye's syndrome – Encephalopathy and liver failure associated with viral infection and aspirin consumption

Rigler's sign of pneumoperitoneum AKA Rigler's sign AKA Rigler sign AKA Double wall sign – x-ray sign where air present on both sides of the bowel wall suggesting pneumoperitoneum and intra-luminal gas/air

Robinson drain – plastic surgical drain that retains its shape (see Jackson-Pratt drain and Penrose drain)

Ryles tube – nasogastric tube or NG tube (typically used to drain)

Sacculi vermibus AKA 'bag of worms' – varicocoele

Sago spleen AKA Fontanus spleen – Splenic amyloidosis where amyloid is deposited in Malpighian corpuscles

Saturday night palsy – palsy of the radial nerve with wrist drop due to prolonged axillary pressure when collapsed with axillae on chair handles

Schamroth Sign AKA Endocarditis clubbing – other causes of clubbing are typicfally repiratory (chronic lung disease), cardiac (cyanotic heart disease), GI (cirrhosis, inflammatory bowel disease, lymphoma). Unilateral clubbing can be associated with hemiplegia and vascular lesions

Scheuermann's disease AKA Scheuermann's Kyphosis AKA Juvenile Kyphosis

Scrofula AKA King's evil AKA Mycobacterial cervical lymphadenitis (see also collar-stud abscess and Ghon focus)

Sims' position, AKA lateral recumbent position – patient laying on one side with upper hip and knee flexed and straight on the side that the patient is lying down

Sister Mary Joseph sign/nodule/node – Palpable umbilical lesion or 'bruising' / ecchymosis suggesting malignant metastasis die to a pelvic or abdominal primary (possibly due to lymphatic spread alongside an obliterated or remnant umbilial vein)

Smead-Jones Closure Suture AKA 'Far-and-Near' technique – Each closure comprises of alternating far and near sutures perpendicular to the fascial tissues being closed

Spinster's claw AKA Ulnar claw – Ulnar nerve injury at wrist, typically seen at rest. The higher up the arm the injury, the less the claw effect as the ulnar nerve also supplies the medial half of the flexor digitorum profundus muscle, AKA 'The Ulnar Paradox', or 'the closer to the Paw, the worse the Claw'

Staghorn calculus – Triple phosphate renal tract stone. Note radio-opaque stones are oxalate (seen in hypercalciuria with laminated black stones on pathology), cystine (inherited conditions or aminoaciduria) and majority of staghorn calculi whereas urate (uric acid) is radio-lucent. Approximately sixty percent of renal stones are radiopaque

Surgical glove port – Cost-effective port system (using a surgical glove) in Single Incision Laparoscopic Surgery (SILS)

Swan-Ganz Catheter– Pulmonary Artery Catheter

Tinel's sign – percussion over a nerve demonstrates irritation due to compression, classical example of median nerve in carpal tunnel syndrome (similar to Hoffmann sign AKA Patel's sign AKA Trotter-Davies sign, related to Phalen's test)

Trendelenburg gait AKA Gluteus medius lurch – Gait abnormality due to abductor muscle (gluteus medius and gluteus minimus) weakness, typically seen with a superior gluteal nerve lesion or in L5 radiculopathy seen in poliomyelitis

Trendelenburg position – supine position with head down to 15-30 degrees used in surgery to gain better access to the pelvis and its organs, or to assist in the management of shock, or as part of the modified-Valsalva manoeuvre. The 'Reverse Trendelenburg' is the opposite to the Trendelenburg where the feet are 15-30 degrees lower

Trendelenburg's sign – clinical tests to asses weakness in the hip abductor muscles (gluteus medius and gluteus minimus)

Trendelenburg Test AKA Brodie-Trendelenburg test – (for varicose vein incompetence, see Vascular section)

TURP Syndrome – Seen after the TURP procedure with confusion, hypotension, occasionally chest pain and notably hyponatraemia on blood tests (<120 mmol/L)). Due to intravascular volume overload, dilutional hyponatraemia and intracellular oedema. Can be treated with frusemide if all other sources for symptoms are excluded

Wunderlich syndrome – condition of renal haemorrhage or angiomyolipoma with middle-to-large vessel vasculitis and or thrombosis e.g. renal thrombosis or cerebral haemorrhage. Comprises of Lenk's triad: (1)Flank mass, (2)Flank pain, (3)Hypovolaemic shock

Volkmann's contracture AKA Volkmann's ischaemic contracture – claw hand or foot associated with non-infective causes (e.g. compartment syndrome)

Valsalva manoeuvre – exhaling against a closed glottis

Venturi mask – Fixed performance mask, interchangeable valve, based on Venturi effect

Virchow's node AKA Troisier's sign AKA sentinel node AKA signal node – palpable left supraclavicular fossa lymph node representing intra-abdominal cancer

Von Hippel-Lindau disease – angiomatosis (cavernous hemangiomas), phaeochromocytoma, renal cell carcinoma, haemangioblastomas, pancreatic cysts (pancreatic serous cystadenoma), endolymphatic sac tumor, and bilateral papillary cystadenomas of the epididymis, broad ligament of the uterus. Type 1 VHL typically has CNS, eye, pancreas and renal tumours and Type 2 is associated with several tumours including phaeochromocytomas

Wallenberg syndrome AKA Lateral medullary syndrome – acute infarction of vasculature to the lateral medulla oblongata; typically, the intracranial portion of the vertebral artery followed by PICA and it's branches. Presents with (1) Vertigo/ Diplopia (2) Horner's (3) Hoarseness due to ipsilateral bulbar weakness

WHO Surgical Safety Checklist – 19 point checklist

designed to improve worldwide surgical safety aimed to decrease errors and adverse events, and increase teamwork and communication in surgery

Ziehl-Neelsen stain – for Mycobacterium (avium, bovis, leprae, tuberculosis)

19.   OESOPHAGUS

Boerhaave / Oesophageal Rupture

Anderson's Triad – Likely abdominal oesophageal rupture: (1)Abdominal rigidity, (2) Subcutaneous emphysema, (3)Raised respiration rate

Boerhaave syndrome – spontaneous oesophageal rupture (usually vertical, rarely transverse) First reported case by Herman Boerhaave, a Dutch physician, described the case of Barron Wassenaer, the Grand Admiral of Holland (in 1724) who died after a large meal and a self-prescribed emetic. Autopsy revealed the rare finding of a transverse oesophageal tear

Hamman's sign of pneumomediastinum AKA (mistakenly as) Hammond's sign AKA (mistakenly as) or Hammond's crunch – praecordial crunching noise in conjunction with heart beat due to mediastinal emphysaema

Mackler's Triad Likely thoracic oesophageal rupture: – (1)Subcutaneous Emphysema, (2)Lower Thoracic Chest

Pain, (3)Vomiting

Mallory–Weiss syndrome AKA Mallory-Weiss Tear AKA Gastro-oesophageal laceration syndrome – laceration at GOJ, lower oesophagus or upper stomach due to vomiting. Typically presents as haemataemsis

Naclerio V sign – radiographic sign of pneumomediastinum where one limb of the V is air between the parietal pleura and the medial left hemi-diaphragm. The other limb of the V is mediastinal air at the left lower mediastinal border.

Spinnaker sign AKA Angel Wing Sign AKA Thymic Spinnaker-Sail Sign – pneumomediastinum in children where air is seen tracking around the thymus

Other radiographic features of pneumomediastinum – 1. Ring-around-the-Artery Sign (Right Pulmonary Artery), 2. Continuous diaphragm sign, 3. Pneumopericardium, 4. Continuous left hemidiaphragm sign, 5. Extrapleural air sign 6. V sign at the confluence of brachiocephalic veins

Oesophageal Pathology

Achalasia AKA 'oesophageal Hirschsprung's disease' AKA achalasia cardiae, AKA cardiospasm AKA esophageal aperistalsis – Oesophageal motility disorder with incomplete relaxation at the lower esophageal sphincter and smooth muscle peristaltic dysfunction. Radiology shows 'birds-beak' or 'rats-tail' sign. Here there are ganglion cells changes at Auerbach's plexus, located between the inner circular and outer longitudinal layers of muscle. In oesophagus, Auerbach's plexus is mainly motor, whereas Meissner's plexus (under the mucosa deep to the muscularis mucosae) is mainly sensory. In the oesophagus, peristalisis is (1) Fast and (2) motor neuronal activity is predominantly free of afferent sensory input, Meissner's plexus is typically absent. As a result, Ganglion cell changes are identified in muscle/ muscularis and not an epithelial biopsy. This contrasts Hirschsprung's disease (see below) where a mucosal biopsy demonstrates absent in Meissner's plexus (and also absent Auerbach's plexus in the muscular layer). Treated by Heller Cardiomyotomy. Please see Hirschsprung's disease below. Can be associated with epiphrenic diverticula and no gastric air bubble due to poor air entry via lower oesophageal sphincter. Eckardt symptom score is used to grade Achalasia: dysphagia frequency, regurgitation, and chest pain, plus the extent of weight loss) with a maximum of 12. In the early stages there is 'vigorous' muscle contraction on manometry ('vigorous achalasia'), however this drops with time

Bird's beak AKA Parrot's beak sign AKA rat's tail sign – radiological sign for achalasia

Chicago Classification of Oesophageal Dysmotility and Achalasia – Type I (Classic Achalasia, Absence of Peristalsis and no pressure, high relax presure), Type II (Absence of Peristalsis, panoesophageal pressure >30mmHg, high relax pressure), Type III (Absence of Peristalsis, >2 spastic contractions, high relax presure)

Barrett's oesophagus – defined by the squamo-columnar junction being (typically more than 3 cm) above the gastro-oesophageal junction and therefore columnar epithelium lining the distal oesophagus. Macroscopically 'salmon pink' features. 30x increased risk of oesophageal adenocarcinoma. Associated with p53 over-expression but negatively associated with H Pylori status. Terms to use by the Montreal Classification:

<3cm is lower cancer risk
ESOM: Endoscopically suspected oesophageal metaplasia
GM+: Gastric Metaplasia
SIM+: Specialised Intestinal Metaplasia

HALO – Radiofrequency Ablation Technique for Barrett's Oesophagus

Prague Criteria:
C: Cardial folds - circumferential Barrett's distance
M: Cardial folds - Most proximal Barrett's Tongue

Romagnoli-Gutschow-Collard (Brussels) Classification of Barrett's adenocarcinomas

type I: short oesophagus, tumour extending over the GOJ;
type II: short oesophagus, tumour not involving the GOJ;
type III: normal length oesophagus, tumour extending over the GOJ, > 3 cm metaplastic area;
type IV: normal length oesophagus, tumour not involving the GOJ, > 3 cm metaplastic area;
type V: normal length oesophagus, tumour centered on the GOJ, < 3 cm metaplastic area.

Seattle Biopsy Protocol for Barrett's – For high-grade dysplasia where 4-quadrant jumbo biopsies are taken every cm for the detection of early adenocarcinoma

Vienna classification – epithelial neoplasia of the digestive tract, used to classify dysplasia in Barrett's oesophagus

Corkscrew oesophagus – Diffuse oesophageal spasm

Diverticulae (Oesophageal) – (a)True (all layers) vs False (mucosa and submucosa), (b) traction (external pulling forces) vs pulsion (intraluminal pressure), (c)location (Upper, Middle, Lower). Both Zenker and Killian-Jamieson diverticulae are false, pulsion and upper

Howel–Evans syndrome AKA Tylosis with oesophageal cancer (TOC) – autosomal dominant condition associated with RHBDF2 gene presenting with hyperkeratosis of the hands and soles of the feet and also associated with oesophageal cancer. Different and unrelated to the term Tylosis associated with the skin condition Diffuse nonepidermolytic palmoplantar keratoderma AKA Unna–Thost disease AKA Unna–Thost keratoderma

Nutcracker oesophagus – Hypercontracting oesophagus

Plummer–Vinson syndrome AKA Paterson–Brown–Kelly syndrome AKA Sideropenic Dysphagia – Increases risk of Squamous Cell Carcinoma of (1) Oesophagus (2) Pharynx. It comprises of:

(a) Dysphagia, (b) iron deficiency anaemia (can have koilonychia) (c) glossitis (d) cheilosis (angular cheileitis) and (e) oesophageal webs, (f) splenomegaly

Sigmoid Oesophagus – Megaoesophagus in Chagas' disease

Zenker diverticulum AKA pharyngeal pouch – False pseudodiverticulum (as all layers of the oesophagus are not present), Pulsion Upper, Diverticula in the posterior midline through the hypopharynx, proximal to the upper oesophageal sphincter between the thyropharyngeus and cricopharyngeus muscles (AKA Killian's dehiscence AKA

Killian's triangle. Symptoms of regurgitation, dysphagia, halitosis, globus sensation. Related to Killian-Jamieson diverticula, also false, pulsion, upper and Killian dehiscence-based, but are smaller (<1.5cm) and rarely symptomatic. Typically present in >70 yr olds

Tertium law – secundum tertium, middle third of oesophagus squamous cell carcinoma more likely, tertium tertium, lower third of oesophagus more likely adenocarcinoma

Oesophageal Operations

Akiyama procedure – srtomach tubulizing and retrosternal route.

Egger AKA Sabre slash incision – Left thoracoabdominal incision for oesophagectomy

Ivor-Lewis 'classic two-stage' (2 incision, laparotomy + thoracotomy) oesophagogastrectomy – (a)Laparotomy/Laparoscopy, mobilisation of stomach, lymph node dissection, feeding Jejunostomy. (b) Thoracotomy/ Thoracoscopy, mobilisation of oesophagus, lymph node dissection→ anastomosis. Lower leak, stricture and aspiration. See Lewis-Tanner procedure below

Kirschner Procedure – Oesophageal stricture procedure with oesophagectomy and gastric mobilisation to the the neck through a presternal skin tunnel. Gastric fundal anastomosis to a proximally divided cervical oesophagus. The distal oesophageal remnant proximally sutured in the neck and its intra-abdominal segment anastomosed to the jejunum with a Roux-en-Y anastomosis. Can also be used for palliative oesophageal cancer.

Klopp Procedure – cervical oesophagostomy

Lewis-Tanner operation – Oesophagogastrectomy similar to the Ivor-Lewis procedure but with a right thoracotomy exclusively

McKeown 'classic three-stage'(3 incision, laparotomy, thoracotomy, neck incision) oesophagogastrectomy – (a) Thoracotomy/Thoracoscopy, mobilisation of oesophagus, lymph node dissection, thoracic duct ligation. This procedure utilises a posterior mediastinal route. (b)Laparotomy/Laparoscopy, mobilisation of stomach, lymph node dissection, feeding Jejunostomy. (c) Cervical incision→ anastomosis. Some consider less local recurrence, easier management of anastomotic leaks at the neck, smaller thoracotomy as neck incision is the site of anastomosis

Orringer procedure – (typically palliative) oesophagectomy with no thoracotomy, abdominal oesophageal resection with direct stomach anastomosis or stomach tube anastomosis

Postlethwait procedure – (typically palliative) similar to the Orringer procedure, oesophagectomy with isoperistaltic stomach tube anastomosis, utilises the Lortat-Jacob's technique to release the oesophagus (where it is used for anti-reflux surgery)

Sweet Left Thoracoabdominal Oesophagectomy AKA Sweet-Churchill procedure (using Sabre slash incision) (contemporary thoracic oesophagectomies include Ohsawa technique and its modification by Garlock and also by Carter. Other techniques by Marshall and Adams & Phemister)

Transhiatal oesophagogastrectomy (2 incision, laparotomy + neck incision) – (a)Laparotomy/Laparoscopy, mobilisation of stomach, lymph node dissection, feeding Jejunostomy, hiatus is widened and mediastinal oesophagus is mobilized. (b) Cervical incision, cervical oesophagus mobilised, upper mediastinum dissected, oesophagus resection and stomach conduit brought up→ anastomosis

Ware-Garrett-Pickrell Procedure – cervical oesophagostomy

Oesophageal Symptoms

Globus hystericus – fullness in the oesophagus not associated with dysphagia

Dysphagia Liquids – Achalasia or Motor Disorder

Dysphagia Solids – mechanical compression (external or internal)

Dysphagia Liquids and Solids – Motor Disorder or late stage mechanical compression

20. PAEDIATRIC

Barbette Disease AKA Barbette-Wilson Disease AKA Intussusception – self-telescoping or invaginating bowel, the invaginator is the 'intussusceptum' and the invaginatee is the 'intussuscipiens'. Typically presents with bowel obstruction between 6-18 months with "blackcurrant jelly' stool. Occurs in 1-in-400 to 1-in-500 patients, most commonly are ileo-colic, treatment can initially be reduction by air enema and if unsuccessful surgery. Can originate at a 'lead point' in the abdomen, for example lymphoid changes due to enlarged Peyer's patches, Henoch–Schönlein purpura or a Meckel's diverticulum. (See Dance's sign). 30% (or a third) have a 'classical' presentation triad of (i)Severe cyclical colic/ abdominal pain, (ii)Bile-stained vomiting and (iii)blackcurrant jelly rectal bleeding. 30% may demonstrate the classical 'sausage-shaped' abdominal mass or 'doughnut'/ target sign on transverse view ultrasound or the pseudo-kidney sign on longitudinal view ultrasound. 80% can be treated with hydrostatic reduction

Bell's Staging Criteria for Necrotizing Enterocolitis – I-Suspected, II-Definite, IIIa-shock, IIIb-perforation

Bochdalek hernia – AKA Back-dalech defect in the posteriorlateral area of the diaphragm (see Morgagni hernia)

Calder Disease AKA Calder Ogle Disease AKA Gastroschisis – abdominal organs outside the abdomen but without the visceral peritoneum or umbilical cord (see Exomphalos below)

Dance's sign of intussusception – abdominal retraction at the right lower quadrant

Double bubble sign – radiological sign typically seen in duodenal atresia representing dilatation of the proximal duodenum and stomach. In Jejunal atresia, a triple bubble/ multiple bubble is seen (double bubble with air in the jejunum also). Single bubble is seen in pyloric stenosis

Hirschprung's Disease – congenital aganglionic length of colon, pathology commences at anus extending upwards. Presentation is bowel obstruction and failure to pass meconium. Classical conical appearance of colon on abdominal contrast radiograph (e.g. barium enema). in a segment of the colon. Absent ganglion cells (derived from the neural crest) in the myenteric smooth muscle (Auerbach) plexus and submucosal (Meissner) plexus (intrinsic innervation as extrinsic innervation is autonomic). Affected segment tonically contracted with histology revealing increased acetylcholinesterase activity. (Of note the Megacolon condition in Chagaz disease resulting from Trypanosoma cruzi has been suggested to derive from its effects of Auerbach's plexus). Several 'pull-through' procedures to treat it have been described. These include the Swenson, Soave and Duhamel procedures. Please see Achalasia above. In Hirschprung's disease there is loss of the rectoanal inhibitory reflex (internal sphincter relaxation and external sphincter contraction following rectal distension AKA 'rectal sampling gate for solids and gases'). This also occurs in low anterior resections (though the reflex returns), progressive systemic sclerosis and Chagas disease.

Henoch–Schönlein purpura AKA IgA vasculitis AKA anaphylactoid purpura AKA purpura rheumatica AKA Schönlein–Henoch purpura – vasculoptahy with skin changes and typically renal dysfunction in children. Likely on the clinical spectrum of Berger's disease

Holliday-Segar Method of caloric and electrolyte replacement –

Works for both kcal and ml of fluid

(First 10) 1-10 kg: 100 kcal/kg/day
(Second 10) 11-20 kg: 50 kcal/kg/day, Cumulative=1500
(Remainder) >20 kg: 20 kcal/kg/day, Cumulative=1500+ xkgx20

Also for fluid replacement/ hr

Up to 10 kg: 4 mls/kg/hr
From 10 - 20 kg: 2 mls/kg, Cumulative =60mls/hr
>20 kg: 1 ml/kg for every kg after, Cumulative=60mls + xkg

Electrolytes: Na+ 3 mEq per 100 kcal/day, K+ 2 mEq per 100 kcal/day, Cl 2 mEq per 100 kcal/day

Keyes sign AKA pneumoscrotum– Could be from perforation, fourniers gangrene, surgery, infection in peritoneum or retroperitoneum incuding incarcerated hernias in neonates

Knudson's 'two-hit' (or 'multiple-hit') **Hypothesis** – multiple mutations are required for a proto-oncogene to lead to cancer, the classical example being Retinoblastoma

Ladd's bands – congenital peritoneal bands seen in intestinal malrotation, typically between an abnormally positioned caecum to peritoneum and liver

Ladd's procedure for intestinal malrotation – division of Ladd's bands, reduction of volvulus if present, appendicectomy and gastropexy

MACE AKA Malone antegrade continence enema AKA **Malone procedure** – appendix used as a conduit for antegrade enema

Meckel's diverticulum AKA Meckel-Hildanus diverticulum – a true bowel diverticulum (all-layers) vestigial remnant of the omphalomesenteric duct (AKA vitelline duct AKA yolk stalk). Rule of 2's: presents under 2yr old, 2% symptomatic, occurs in 2% of the population, 2:1 male:female, typically within 2 feet of the ileoceacal valve, typically 2 inches in length, two-thirds have ectopic mucosa, two types of heterotopic mucosa (gastric and pancreatic), 2 main complications of obstruction and bleeding. Presentation can be painless haematochezia. Can be the route of the stone in gallstone ileus. Can be participate in Littre's hernia

Mitrofanoff procedure AKA Mitrofanoff appendicovesicostomy – appendix used as a conduit for bladder drainage

Monti procedure – Segment of GI Tract used as a conduit for bladder drainage

Morgagni hernia – AKA Morg-Anterior Defect in the

anterior para-sternal area of the diaphragm. Also T8 (Cava CavEight), T10 (Oesophagus), T12 (Aorta, Aortwelve), (see Bochdalek hernia)

Oesophagoscopes in children: Storz rigid bronchoscope, Negus instrument, Chevalier-Jackson instrument

Pare Disease AKA Pare-Mery Disease AKA Exomphalos AKA Omphalocele/ Omphalocoele – abdominal organs outside the abdomen enclosed in visceral peritoneum with the umbilical cord (see Gastroschisis above)

Pneumatosis cystoides intestinalis – intramural bowel gas seen in necrotising enterocolitis

Ramstedt pyloromyotomy AKA Stiles-Ramstedt pyloromyotomy – operation for Pyloric stenosis (not unusual for pylorus to be lengthened, but this is not a 'pyloroplasty'). This presents biochemically as Dehydration with (1)Metabolic alkalosis (2)Hypochloraemia, (3)Hypokalaemia, (4)Hypercapnea (5)typically Hyponatraemia. 'Single bubble' may be seen on x-ray

(1)Vomiting acid (hydrochloric acid) results in alkalosis
(2)Low blood chloride level decreases renal bicarbonate excretion so the alkalosis is uncorrected alkalosis
(3)Vomiting fluid decreases circulating volume so there is secondary hyperaldosteronism (holding Na+ and losing K+ in the urine, hence hypokalaemia
(4)respiratory compensation to the metabolic alkalosis with hypoventilation an an elevated arterial pCO2 (hypercapnea)

Ribes rubrum faeces AKA redcurrant jelly stools – intussusception

Tongue-Tie AKA Ankyloglossia – decreased tongue tip mobility due to a short and thick lingual frenulum

Tumours in childhood (incidence) – (1)Leukaemias, (2)brain tumours, (3) lymphomas (4th equal) Neuroblastoma & Wilms' tumour

Wilms' tumour – childhood renal neoplasm. 10% bilateral, one third due to deletions in chromosome 11. Can be associated with Genitourinary abnormalities, Hemihypertrophy, Sporadic aniridia (1%). Associated syndrome include WAGR syndrome (Wilms' tumour, aniridia, genitourinary malformations, mental retardation), Denys-Drash syndrome (Wilms' tumour, nephropathy, genital abnormalities) and Beckwith-Wiedemann syndrome (Wilms', overgrowth, macroglossia, omphalocoele)

VACTERL syndrome – Vertebral, Ano-rectal, Cardiac, Tracheo-oEsophageal, Renal and Radial Limb anomalies

21. PANCREAS

Atlanta classification of acute pancreatitis – (i) Mild (no organ failure, no local complications), (ii) Moderate (organ failure <48hrs +/- local complications), (iii) Severe (Persistent organ failure >48hrs). Organ failure primarily cardiac, respiratory and renal. Local compolications are fluid, pseudo-cysts, necrosis, pleural effusions

Balthazar score – CT scoring system of Pancreatitis severity (A-E) scoring respectively (0-4), then added to pancreatic necrosis score (0, <30, 30-50, >50%) scoring respectively (0-6). Added together they achive a maximum of 10 corresponding to the the CT severity index (CTSI)

Cullen sign (peri-umbilical ecchymosis discoloration secondary to haemoperitoneum)

Deathstalker Pancreatitis AKA Israeli or Palestine yellow scorpion pancreatitis AKA Omdurman scorpion pancreatitis AKA Naqab desert scorpion pancreatitis – Levantine scorpion (Leiurus quinquestriatus) whose venomous bite can induce pancreatitis

Grey-Turner sign (red-brown/ ecchymosis in flanks resulting from retroperitoneal haematoma)

Lundh's test of pancreatic exocrine function – sampling of duodenal contents for enzymatic activity (amylase, trypsin, lipase) 2hours after a meal of carbohydrate, protein and fat

Mallet-Guy sign of pancreatitis – pain on palpation of the epigastrium and left subcostal region

Pancreas Dermatitis – Erythematous skin nodules, typically on extensor surfaces (<1cm) and associated with polyarthropathy

Modified Glasgow or Glasgow-Imrie Criteria:
(P)PaO2< 7.9kPa or <60mmHg
(A)Age > 55 years
(N)Neutrophils (WBC > 15x10^9/L)
(C)Calcium < 2 mmol/L
(R)Renal function: Urea > 16 mmol/L
(E)Enzymes LDH > 600 IU/L
(A)Albumin < 32g/L (serum)
(S)Sugar (blood glucose) > 10 mmol/L

Where Mortality:
0 to 2: 2%
3 to 4: 15% (3 or above is considered severe pancreatitis requiring HDU/ITU)
5 to 6: 40%
7 to 8: 100%

Trinidad Thick-tailed Scorpion Pancreatitis – Trinidadian scorpion (Tityus trinitatis) whose venomous bite can induce pancreatitis

Chronic Pancreatitis

Beger Procedure – Duodeno-Pancreatic Duct preserving head of pancreas resection

Berne-Farkas procedure AKA Berne-Büchler-Farkas procedure – Duodenal preserving head of pancreas resection

Frey's procedure AKA Frey-Smith Procedure – Duodenal preserving head of pancreas resection, coring out diseased section of pancreas and lateral pancreaticojejunostomy (LRLPJ) to the pancreatic duct (side-to-side). A type of local head resection with lateral pancreaticojejunostomy, LR-LPJ

Ho-Frey procedure AKA Frey-Ho procedure – pancreatic head core excavation and core drainage with Roux-en-Y pancreaticojejunostomy

Hamburg Modification of Izbicki – Coring out pancreatic head and V Pancreaticojejunostomy

Izbicki procedure – Coring out pancreatic head and V pancreaticojejunostomy, a type of local head resection with lateral pancreaticojejunostomy, LR-LPJ

Kausch procedure – pancreaticojejunostomy

Kutup procedure – Longitudinal 'V' excision

Link procedure – pancreaticojejunostomy

Partington-Rochelle procedure–pancreaticojejunostomy

Puestow procedure AKA Puestow-Gillesby procedure –

side-to-side pancreaticojejunostomy

Whipple procedure AKA Kausch-Whipple procedure – Resection of head of pancreas, duodenum, gastric antrum and gallbladder

Whipple II procedure AKA pylorus-preserving pancreaticoduodenectomy (PPPD) AKA Traverso-Longmire procedure

22. SKIN

Basalioma AKA Basal cell carcinoma – Shiny, Pearly papule or nodule, rolled edge, ubmilicated centre with telangectasias VS SCC which are typically in older patients, everted edge, hyperkeratotic, ulcerating and seen in immunosuppressed or transplant patients. Include Fibroepithelioma of Pinkus and Rodent ulcer AKA Jacob's ulcer

Blaschko's lines – Cutaneous mosaicism, can be associated with linear atrophoderma of Moulin

Blueberry lesion AKA Keratocanthoma AKA Molluscum Sebaceum AKA self-healing' squamous cell carcinoma – sun/UV exposure condition, red with a central punctum/ hyperkeratitic core. Typically in the elderly that is histologically considered to be in the same/similar class as squamous cell carcinoma (SCC) although is not formally 'pre-malignant', also seen in Muir-Torre Syndrome. Several types including (i)Ferguson-Smith Syndrome (multiple-self healing lesions), (i)Generalized eruptive keratoacanthoma of Grzybowski, (iii)Giant-type, (iv) Solitary/ Subungal type. Treatments may include Mohs surgery

Breslow depth/ level – skin cancer invasion depth to stage (I-V) melanoma disease (used typically in conjunction with Clark's level, see below).Covers <0.75mm to >3mm

Bowen's disease AKA squamous cell carcinoma in situ – typically seen on women's lower legs (60-85%) or builders, large, hyperchromatic nuclei. They can present with raised edges. When associated with burns or non-healing ulcers are called Marjolin's ulcers

Café au lait macules (CALMs) – typically seen in von Recklinghausen's disease (Neurofibromatosis type 1), Neurofibromatosis type 2 and several other conditions including: Ash leaf spots & Tuberous sclerosis, Ataxia telangiectasia, Basal cell nevus syndrome, Bloom syndrome, Chédiak–Higashi syndrome, Fanconi anaemia, Gaucher disease, Hunter syndrome, Legius syndrome, Maffucci syndrome, McCune-Albright syndrome 'coast of Maine', Multiple mucosal neuroma syndrome, Silver-Russell syndrome, Watson syndrome

Clark's level – skin cancer invasion depth to stage (I-V) melanoma disease (used typically in conjunction with Breslow depth if very thin (<1 mm) melanomas. Based on invasion of epidermis, dermis or subcutaneous fat

Chloasma faciei AKA Melasma AKA Mask of Pregnancy

Cylindroma AKA 'TurbanTumour' – condition of multiple scalp tumours that are a variant of eccrine spiradenomas

Dercum's disease AKA Anders disease AKA Adiposis Dolorosa AKA Fatty Tissue Rheumatism AKA Juxta-Articular Adiposis Dolorosa AKA Lipomatosis Dolorosa

AKA Morbus Dercum's – (1) painful lipomas (multiple), (2) obesity, (3) fatigue and weakness and (4) Neuropsychiatric diseases, e.g. depression and or dementia and or epilepsy. Autosomal dominant and female to male ratio in 20:1. It is related to (but not the same as) Madelung's disease AKA Benign Symmetrical Lipomatosis, typically seen in alcoholics as a metabolic disorder of body fats

Duhring's disease AKA Dermatitis herpetiformis – skin rash with watery blisters not caused by herpes virus but looking similar. Associated with Coeliac disease, HLA-DQ2 haplotype, particularly in northern Europeans and northern Indians.

Erythema Types and Diseases

Ab igne AKA Laptop thigh syndrome AKA Hot water bottle rash AKA granny's tartan AKA toasted skin syndrome – reticulated hypermelanosis with erythema associated with close persistent infa-red skin exposure (see Kangri cancer)

Chronicum migrans – Lyme disease

Elevatum diutinum – Immune diseases, Coeliac disease and paraproteinaemias such as monoclonal IgA gammopathy

Gyratum repens AKA 'repeating rings' – Malignancy

Induratum – Tuberculosis

Infectiosum AKA 'Slapped cheeks' – Parvovirus B19

Multiforme – 'Target lesions' due to Herpes Simplex, Mycoplasma, Orf

Marginatum – Acute glomerulonephritis, Drugs and classically Rheumatic Fever

Necrolytic migratory erythema – Pancreatic islet cell carcinoma

Nodosum AKA Subacute migratory panniculitis of

Vilanova and Piño – Typically on shins but could be on abdomen e.g. umbilicus, Can be associated with Inflammatory Bowel Disease, Leprosy, Streptococcus, Sarcoidosis, Sulphonamides, Tuberculosis and others

Erythroplasia de Queyrat (subtype of Bowen's disease) – squamous-cell carcinoma in situ of the glans penis, inner prepuce (foreskin) or vulva

Fitzpatrick skin type AKAS Fitzpatrick phototyping scale – Classification of skin colour as a predictor for categorising sun-exposed cancer risk (I[fair] – VI [dark])

Glomus tumour AKA Glomangioma – Rare tumour of the nail or fingertip

Gorlin syndrome AKA Gorlin–Goltz syndrome AKA Nevoid basal-cell carcinoma syndrome (NBCCS) AKA basal-cell nevus syndrome AKA multiple basal-cell carcinoma syndrome

Hartnup disease AKA Hartup disorder – pellagra-like dermatosis

Hebra-Kaposi disease AKA 'Moon Child' AKA Xeroderma pigmentosum – autosomal recessive DNA gyrase disease associated with XP gene resulting in multiple basal cell carcinomas (basaliomas) or other skin cancers (the term 'Moon Child' is because patients should never be exposed to light)

Henoch–Schönlein purpura AKA anaphylactoid purpura AKA Purpura rheumatic – IgA Systemic Vasculitis most typically in the skin but also other organs (such as the kidney)

Hutchinson's freckle AKA Lentigo maligna – radial

growth and no vertical growth, carcinoma in situ, non-invasive (3rd most common type of melanoma, Most common Superficial Spreading (multiple colours, brown, black, red, blue, white), 2nd Nodular (worst prognosis), 4th Acral). Typically on cheeks

Kangri cancer AKA Neve syndrome – Squamous-cell carcinoma of the skin found in Kashmir, associated with the kangri undergarment and erythema ab igne

Klippel-Trenaunay-Weber syndrome –Comprises of (1) port-wine (naevus flammeus) stains, (2)varicose veins (3)limb gigantism (bone and soft tissue hypertrophy)

Langer's lines – morphological/developmental cleavage lines

Lupus Agricolae AKA Seborrhoeic Keratoses AKA Basal Cell Papilloma – Pigmented lesions in sun exposed areas

Lupus Insecta AKA Dermatofibroma AKA Histiocytoma – Cutanous response to insect bite or minor trauma

Lupus Pernio – Cutaneous Sarcoid

Lupus Vulgaris – Cutaneous TB

Marjolin ulcer – SCC associated with burns or non-healing ulcers

Merkel cell carcinoma – rare neuroendocrine tumour noted arising from sun/ UV exposed areas of the skin, if found Oat cell carcinoma of the lung needs to be investigated as it has similar skin metastases
Mole AKA melanocytic nevus – 3 locations (i) junctional

[of epidermis and dermis] (ii) compound [junctional + intra-dermal] (iii) intra-dermal. Types: Acquired, Blue, Congenital, Dysplastic (Clarke), Intra-mucosal, Ita & Ota (skin and shoulders), Mongolian spot (Blue, large, seen in Asians), Recurrent, Spitz (children)

Molluscum sebaceum AKA keratokanthoma – Typically self-limiting/ self-resolving condition with central necrosis and ulceration. Histologically similar to squamous cell carcinoma. Can leave a scar. Typically resected as could be SCC

Mohs micrographic surgery – for excision of advanced BCCs and SCCs

Pellagra – dermatitis from chronic lack of niacin (vitamin B3 or vitamin PP). Can be present in carcinoid syndrome and protein metabolism disorders. It has an association with dementia (though not with carcinoid). Can be clinically similar to Hartnup disease. Presents with 4 D's: diarrhoea, dermatitis, dementia, death

Port-wine stain AKA Naevus Flammeus AKA Firemark – 'birth mark' due to vascular capillary anomaly. Can be seen in several syndromes such as as Sturge–Weber syndrome and Klippel–Trénaunay–Weber syndrome (incidentally both of which have Weber as an eponym)

'Seven year itch' AKA scabies – Sarcoptes scabiei infection

Solar keratosis AKA Actinic keratosis – most common pre-malignant skin lesion in light skin

Stewart-Treves syndrome – rare angiosarcoma that can be found on face or scalp and associated with chronic lymphoedema after axillary dissection

Squamous Cell Carcinoma – Majority on head and neck, non-healing hyper-keratotic sun-exposed area ulcer

Stork bite AKA Naevus flammeus nuchae – capillary malformation causing birthmark on back of neck and head (usually temporary)

Sturge–Weber syndrome AKA Encephalotrigeminal Angiomatosis – congenital disorder of: (1) Skin, port-wine stains, (2) Brain (angiomas), (3) seizures, (4) eyes, galucomas, (5) mental retardation. 3 types exist: Type 1, eye and brain involvement, Type 2, Facial skin and eye involvement and Type 3, predominantly brain involvement. Sporadic Sturge–Weber syndrome occurs due to a somatic activating mutation of the GNAQ gene

Touraine Solente Gole syndrome – Primary hypertrophic osteoathropathy, hereditary primary pachydermoperiostosis. Triad of pachydermia (elephant-like skin), periostosis and acropachia with clubbing

Voight's lines – skin area boundaries supplied by one cutaneous nerve

Vulcano lesion AKA Dermatofibroma AKA Fibrous Histiocytoma – Typically from insect bites/ trauma. 'Pinch test': squeezing the lesion on the sides of the 'mini-volcano' demonstrates dimpling of overlying skin.

Zadik's operation – matrisectomy procedure for ingrowing toenails

23. STATISTICS

Akaike information criterion AKA AIC – Quality measure for statistical models, typically in regression

Analysis

Non-parametric with independent and dependent variables

Breslow-Day test for homogeneous association – for a 2 x 2 x Z table, to see if all Z strata have the same OR. If OR is not given, the Cochran-Mantel-Haenszel estimate (below)should be applied. This is because the Cochran-Mantel-Haenszel test presumes homogeneity of treatment effects in all strata. The Breslow-Day tests the homogeneity assumption of Cochran-Mantel-Haenszel, and not relevant for small strata such as pairs. Homogeneity = the conditional relationship of 2 variables is the same level for both at the 3rd

Cochran–Mantel–Haenszel test for repeated tests of independence for matched categorical data to see if the tests are independent (supposes that the effect of the treatment is homogeneous in all strata)

Pearson Chi Square: Categorical Large

Chi Square with Yates' correction for continuity: Categorical Small (<10 or <5 studies)

Fisher's Exact Test: Categorical Small

Paired –

Spearman's rank test AKA Spearman's rank correlation coefficient or Spearman's rho: Ordinal (one sample e.g. of people, or more)

Wilcoxon T AKA Wilcoxon signed-rank test AKA Wilcoxon-Mann-Whitney test: equivalent of paired t-test for non-parametric data, Ordinal (two samples, dependent).

Friedman ANOVA by Ranks: Ordinal (three samples +, dependent)

van Elteren test for nonparametric two-way analysis, a stratified subtype of the Wilcoxon-Mann-Whitney test for comparing two treatments accounting for strata

Unpaired –

Mann-Whitney U test: Ordinal (two samples, independent).

Kruskal-Wallis H test AKA One-way ANOVA on ranks: Ordinal (three samples +, independent)

Kolmogorov-Smirnov test AKA KS-test – asses if two datasets are significantly different making no assumption regarding data distribution

Kendall rank correlation coefficient AKA Kentalls tau: non-parametric equivalent of Pearson's correlation

Parametric AKA Gaussian AKA Normal distribution

Gossett test AKA Student's t-test

Friedman ANOVA

Pearson product-moment correlation coefficient: measure of strength and correlation between two variables

Welch's t-test AKA unequal variances t-test

Z-test – assessing two population means with known variances and large sample size

Bayesian information criterion AKA BIC – Quality measure for a statistical models, typically in regression

Bias – Analytical, Ascertainment, Attrition, Chance, Consent, Delay, Dilution, Exclusion, Funding, Hawthorne effect (observer effect), Observer bias, Publication, Recruitment, Reporting, Resentful demoralisation, Subversion, Technical

Causation

Bradford Hill criteria AKA Hill's criteria for causation –

(1)Strength (effect size)
(2)Consistency (reproducibility)
(3)Specificity
(4)Temporality
(5)Biological gradient
(6)Plausibility
(7)Coherence
(8)Experiment
(9)Analogy

Cox regression AKA proportional hazards regression

Data

(I)Discrete – (a)Nominal/ Categorical (e.g. Blood Group, Gender), (b)Ordinal (orders e.g. 1st, 2nd) (Always NON-PARAMETRIC)

(II)Continuous – (a)Interval (e.g. Temperature), (b)Ratio (interval with an absolute of 0, e.g. height and weight)

Galbraith plot AKA Galbraith's radial plot – demonstrating multiple estimates of one factor with different standard errors

Gray's test for subdistribution hazards – Compares cumulative incidence functions applied for the evaluation of hypotheses of equality of cause-specific cumulative incidence functions between two groups

Greedy Algorithm – algorithmic paradigm used to make optimal 'Greedy' choices for decisions and can be used in matching for propensity scoring (for example Greedy nearest neighbour)

Hosmer–Lemeshow test – test to assess goodness of fit in logistic regression

Kaplan–Meier estimator – non-parametric survival function

Meta-analysis – combined several studies, level 1a evidence is a meta-analysis of randomised controlled trials (RCTS). Random-effects (DerSimonian and Laird) and Fixed-effects analysis. Forest plots are used to demonstrate results. Multiple types: Standard, Diagnostic, Network, Individual Patient and Umbrella. Peto OR (odds ratio) used to describe results

Mallows's Cp – modification of Akaike information criterion utilising ordinary least squares in the special case of Gaussian linear regression

Nulrej 1 – Type I error, rejecting the null hypothesis falsely

Nulacc 2 – Type II error, accepting the null hypothesis falsely

Hazard ratios consider a function of time and are used in survival analysis

Health Performance Scores – These include the: Eastern Cooperative Oncology Group (ECOG), Global Assessment of Functioning (GAF) score, Karnofsky score, Lansky score (children), Zubrod score(used by the WHO)

Screening

UK National Screening Committee 2003
22 criteria spread across: (1) condition, (2) test, (3) treatment, (4) screening programme

Wilson and Junger's (WHO) criteria for screening –

The condition being screened for should be an important health problem
The natural history of the condition should be well understood
There should be a detectable early stage
Treatment at an early stage should be of more benefit than at a later stage
A suitable test should be devised for the early stage
The test should be acceptableIntervals for repeating the test should be determined
Adequate health service provision should be made for the extra clinical workload resulting from screening
The risks, both physical and psychological, should be less than the benefits
The costs should be balanced against the benefits

Studies

Randomised AKA Randomised Control Trials (RCT)– quality assessed by Jadad scale AKA Jadad score

Case-control, good for – Rare disease, multiple risks, minimal loss to follow-up, cheap, reported as OR (odds ratio)

Cohort Studies – time consuming and need large numbers for rare outcomes, but can still look for rare outcomes and less susceptible to recall bias than case control studies, reported as RR (relative risk)

Poisson distributions used for rare events

Weibull distribution – specific subtype of continuous probability distribution

Simpson's paradox AKA Yule–Simpson effect AKA Amalgamation paradox – loss of significance/ trend in individual series when they are combined, in categorical data may need to use the Cochran–Mantel–Haenszel test for repeated tests of independence

24. TRANSPLANT

Cocoon sign – radiological sign of encapsulating peritoneal sclerosis (EPS) on abdominal radiograph

CHIMP – Contraindications to transplantation (absolute)

CJD
HIV (active)
Infection (uncontrolled, sepsis in donor)
Metastases or Malignancy
Past history of malignancy with persistent risk (e.g. melanoma, choriocarcinoma)

Conditions requiring assessment before transplantation (relative): BIPEDAL

Blood pressure
Infection (treated, bacterial, hepatitis B or C, viral hepatitis, risk factors for HIV)
Past history of malignancy with long cancer free period
Elderly age
Diabetes mellitus
Acute Renal Failure

Localised tumours (kidney, prostate)

DRIL – Distal Revascularisation with Interval Ligation used to treat symptomatic av-fistula ischaemic steal syndrome

Fistulas:

Artery-side Venous-side, Artery-side Venous-end (Brescia-Cimino AKA Brescia-Cimino-Appel)
Artery-end Venous-end, Artery-end Venous-side

Machinery murmur – AV fistula murmur continuous throughout cardiac cycle, represents av fistula is working well

Tenckhoff catheter – currently favoured for continuous ambulatory peritoneal dialysis (CAPD) or Acute Peritoneal Dialysis

Trocath catheter – older dialysis catheter

Drug Complications:

5-FU (thymidylate synthase inhibitor) – hand-foot syndrome AKA almar-plantar erythrodysesthesia
Anthracycline (from Streptomyces, topoisomerase II inhibitor) Cardiotoxicity Specifically Doxorubicin Cardiomyopathy
Azathioprine – Lecopaenia, Lymphoma, Blood dyscrasias, TPMT bone marrow suppression
Bleomycin (induction of DNA strand breaks) – induced lung fibrosis
Cyclosporine (Calcineurin inhinitor) – Interstitial Cystitis,

Nephrotoxicity, Gingival Hyperplasia (particularly with calcium channel antagonists, e.g Nifedipine), Hirsutism Cyclosporine and MMF Nephrotoxicity

Cytosine arabinoside AKA Cytarabine (inhibits DNA)– cerebellar toxicity, conjunctivitis, bone marrow suppression

Chemotherapy induced neutropenic enterocolitis (typically ileocaecal area) AKA Typhlitis (specifically the caecum)

Hydroxychloroquine (blocks toll-like receptors and potentiates dendritic antigen presentation to T cells) – Cataracts and retinitis

Methylprednisolone – Diabetes, Obesity, Hypertesnsion

Mycophenolate mofetil (inhibitor of inosine monophosphate dehydrogenase limiting synthesis of guanosine nucleotides, particularly for T- and B-lymphocytes) – Diarrhoea, General GI symptoms, Bone Marrow Suppression (Wight cells)

Methotrexate (antimetabolite of the antifolate type)– Folate deficiency, pulmonary fibrosis and cirrhosis

Sirolimus (Rapamycin) macrolide – Lymphocele, Poor wound healing

Sulfasalazine (inhibition of the cystine-glutamate antiporter) – Oligospermia, thrombocytopenia, leucopenia, haemolytic anaemia

Tacrolimus – Nephrotoxicity, diabetes, hair loss, headaches, tremors

Valganciclovir (1)gingival hypertrophy (2)glossitis (3)nail pigmentation

Vincristine (anti-mitotic and anti-microtubule alkaloid agents) – Deep tendon reflex loss

MACI MATTS (Immunosuppressants)
Metabolite(anti) – Methotrexate, 5FU, Capecitabine
Alkylating – Cyclophosphamide
Calcineurin inhibitor – Cyclosporine, Tacrolimus
Immune antibody – Bevacizumab, Trastuzumab

Micro-Tubule – Vinca Alklaoid, Taxanes
Anthracycline – Doxorubicin
Topoisomerase – Topotecan, Irinotecan
(m)Tor – Sirolimus
Steroids

Graft failure HAVAU– Hyperacute rejection, Acute rejection (within 6 months), arterial stenosis (hypertension and peripheral oedema), venous stenosis (pain and local oedema), Lymphocoele (painless mass), Urinary leak (fever and pain)

Piggyback technique – Utilised in Liver and Cardiac transplants where the transplanted organ is located within the immediate local circulation of the native organ, 'piggybacking' on the native organ

Wisconsin cold storage solution AKA University of Wisconsin solution AKA UW solution – one of the first and most prominent preservation mediums for organ transplantation

25. TRAUMA AND BURNS

APACHE score – Acute Physiology and Chronic Health Evaluation, versions I, II and III exist

Ashrafian Thoracotomy AKA Aztec Thoracotomy – pre-Hospital emergency thoracotomy consisiting of a modified anterior thoracotomy with costochondral release designed to gain rapid access to the pericardium and heart

Ballance's sign of splenic rupture/hematoma – LUQ and left flank percussion dullness with shifting dullness to the RUQ and right flank

Baux score to predict post-burns mortality – BSA + patient's age

Clamshell thoracotomy – swallow incision and thoracotomy exposing mediastinum and lungs bilaterally in trauma situation for emergency care

Bogota bag laparostomy – 3l plastic bag to closure anterior abdominal wall, has the advantage to assess intra-peritoneal contents

Crush syndrome AKA Traumatic Rhabdomyolysis – Muscle crush and ischaemia injury resulting in (1)myoglobin release and (2)hyperkalaemia (3)Other toxic muscle metabolites. Myoglobin can produce renal failure therefore treatment is with Fluid and Sodium Bicarbonate Urine Alkalisation. Diagnostic criteria:

Crush injury to a large mass of skeletal muscle
Sensory & motor disturbance in compressed limbs
Swollen and tense limbs
Myoglobinuria +/- haematuria
Creatine kinase (CK) >1000 U/L (at peak)
Renal pathology with (a)Oliguria (urine output <400 ml/24 hr) (b)Raised Urea and Creatinine, (c)Hyperkalaemia, (d)Hyperuricaemia, (e)Hyperphosphataemia and/or (f)hypocalcaemia

Jordan-Vaughan procedure for duodenal (D1) trauma AKA pyloric exclusion procedure – Primary duodenal repair (duodenorrhaphy)of the duodenal wound, closure of the pylorus through gastrotomy and gastrojejunostomy at the site gastrostomy.

Critchlow Procedure – Roux-en-Y duodenojejunostomy for D2 Trauma or duodenal diverticula

Kocherisation of the duodenum AKA Kocher's manoeuvre – dissection (lateral) of the duodenum (+/- pancreas head) off the retroperitoneum. Can be extended by a Kocher+ manoeuvre AKA Cattell-Brasch manoeuvre toward the right white line of Toldt and subsequently across the small bowel mesenteric root. This begins at begins at the common bile duct and ends at the ligament of Treitz. This exposes the inframesocolic retroperitoneum, IVC, infra-renal aorta, both renal hila, both iliac vessels and superior mesenteric vessels (can be used in Trauma and Vascular Surgery). OF NOTE Its opposite on the LEFT side is the Mattox manoeuvre (also used in traumatology) mobilising left sided abdominal organs to access and control retroperitoneal haematoma. Opposite to Kocher+, it begins at the left sided line of Toldt at the descending colon and extends to the right upper quadrant, thereby freeing the left colon, left kidney, pancreas and spleen

Le Fort fracture classification – For midface fractures

Flagellum Pectus AKA Flail Chest – >2 fractured ribs which move paradoxically during breathing, i.e. sucked in on inspiration and expanded on expiration

Glasgow Coma Score – score of 3-15 points best on eye, motor and verbal functioning used to stratify head trauma

Lund-Browder chart – calculation of percentage burns in children and also in adults, see also Wallace "rule of nines". Also caloric replacement in burns adults: Curreri, Davies and Lilijedahl, Harris Benedict, Ireton-Jones, Toronto Formula. In children: Curreri junior and Galveston

Monro-Kellie Doctrine – The cranium has a fixed volume so that in extra-dural haematoma there is an urgent need to release underlying pressure to prevent damage to other intra-cranial structures

Parkland formula – Fluid replacement in burns: $V(mL) = 4$ x m(kg) x Area(BSA) x 100

Pytherch's POSSUM AKA P-POSSUM – (i) Physiological Factors: Age, Cardiac, ECG report, Respiratory, Blood Pressure, Heart Rate, Coma Scales, Haemoglobin, White Cell Count, Urea, Sodium, Potassium (ii) Operative Factors: Operative Complexity, Multiple

Procedures, Blood Loss, Peritoneal Contamination, Extent of malignant spread, Elective versus emergency surgery

Sennertus syndrome AKA Sennertus-Paré disease – Trauma related diaphragmatic rupture or herniation

Towne view: Skull x-ray that offers better views of the occipital bone and posterior fossa space

Triangulus Salutis AKA Triangle of Safety for Chest Drain Insertion – (1) anterior to mid axillary line (or anterior to Latissimus Dorsi) (2) posterior to pectoral groove (or lateral to pectoralis major) (3) above 5th intercostal space (or at the level of the nipple). Note the axilla is at the apex of this triangle

TRISS AKA Trauma Score-Injury Severity Score – determines trauma survival probability based on the physiologic Revised Trauma Score (RTS) and anatomic Injury Severity Score (ISS)

Wallace 'Rule of Nines' – calculation of percentage burns in adults, see also Lund-Browder chart for children and also in adults

Wallenberg syndrome AKA Lateral medullary syndrome – occlusion/ischaemia to the lateral medulla oblongata, typically intracranial vertebral artery and the posterior inferior cerebellar artery causing VISA symptoms:
V-Vertigo/vestibulocerebellar symptoms
I-Ipsilalteral bulbar symptoms (e.g. dysphagia, dysphonia, dysarthria)
S-Sensory/Stabbing symptoms to ispilatral face and temperature to contralateral face
A-Autonomic dysfuction/Horner's

26. VASCULAR

ABCD2 score – clinical risk of stroke in patients having recently suffered from a transient ischemic attack (TIA), based on : Age, Blood pressure, Clinical features, Duration of TIA, and Presence of diabetes);

Acrocyanosis – Blue discoloration of extremities

Adson Procedure – Scalenectomy without rib resection
Murphy Procedure – removal of first rib

Adson's Test for **Thoracic Outlet Syndrome (TOS)** – radial pulse loss on ipsilateral head rotation during deep inspiration with extended neck. See also Eden's Test, Peete Syndrome, Roos Test and Wright's Test

Positivity can be associated with a cervical rib (subclavian artery can be squashed between the clavicle and rib or band or scalenus anterior). Microemboli due to subclavian post-stenotic dilatation.

If Arterial may cause Raynaud's phenomenon (or secondary Raynaud's) – spasm of hand arteries causing hands to turn white and then blue.

If Venous AKA Paget-Schroetter syndrome or Paget-von Schroetter syndrome – prominent upper body veins that do no collapse on limb elevation

Ashrafian aortic auscultation – auscultation of aorta between the scapulae to assess for a bruit in thoracic aneurysmal disease

Allen's test (modified) – testing patency of radial or ulnar artery. With elevated hand, fingers are clenched and opened whilst either radial artery or ulnar artery are compressed so that the hand slowly blanches. When compression of artery released, the hand should regain normal colour in 5-15s

Amputations:

Ankle:
Syme AKA Symes' amputation – through the ankle joint

Below knee/ Tibial:
Burgess AKA Kendrick-Burgess – Trans-tibial long posterior flap

Robinson AKA Kingsley Robinson – Trans-tibial, skew flap

Brückner – Modified trans-tibial long posterior flap

General:
Teale technique – long and short rectangular flaps
Guillotine technique – circular cut and complete sawing
Racket technique – longitudinal straight with spiral on the sides below

Knee/ Above knee:
Gritti-Stokes – knee disarticulation, oval anterior flap
Mazet – Patella removed and conical stump created
Nellis-van de Water – femoral condyles excised and patella placed at the end of the femur
Sabanajeff – similar to Gritti-Stokes but Patella kept
Youkey – Patella and condyles

Krukenberg procedure AKA Krukenberg operation – conversion of a forearm stump into a pincer formation

Ray 'racket incision' – digital, typically in feet removing the toe and the distal tarsal bone, i.e toe and meta-tarsal

Trans-metatarsal:
LisFranc(k) – base of metatarsal
Chopart – between Navicular-Cuboid and Calcaneus-Talus. Transtarsal

Calcaneus:
Pirogoff
Boyd
LeFort
Günter
Spitzy

Blue toe syndrome – Atherosclerotic plaque rupture in the iliac or femoral arteries

Brearley's rule – if you can feel a vascular pulse (e.g. In a peripheral limb) then you should be able to count it

Buergers Disease AKA Buerger's Disease AKA Thromboangiitis Obliterans – Inflammation and thrombosis of small and medium sized arteries

Buerger's test of arterial sufficiency AKA Rubor of dependency test – raising leg of supine patient to Buerger's angle (where it becomes pale) then dropping it to allow gravity to allow blood flow to leg, whereupon if very hyperaemic or red and takes time to become normal colour (sunset foot) this is a sign of arterial insufficiency. A Buerger's angle <20 degrees represents very severe ischaemia

CHA2DS2–VASc score – Risk of stroke in patients with non-rheumatic atrial fibrillation (AF): Congestive heart failure (or Left ventricular systolic dysfunction) [1], Hypertension (>140/90 mmHg or on medication) [1], Age ≥75 years[2], Diabetes Mellitus [1], Stroke or TIA or thromboembolism (prior) [2], Vascular disease (e.g. peripheral artery disease, myocardial infarction [1], aortic plaque), Age 65–74 years [1], Sex category (i.e. female sex) [1]

Champagne Bottle sign AKA Below-knee Sclerosing Panniculitis AKA Below-knee Lipodermatosclerosis AKA Chronic panniculitis with lipomembranous changes AKA Hypodermitis sclerodermiformis – Seen in obesity associated with Gaiter Ulceration AKA Venous Ulceration

Charcot joint –neuropathic / neurotrophic joint

Chevrier's tap test – venous incompetence, 'transmission down a column'

Cowie's sign – Persistent Sciatic Artery where there are palpable popliteal and/or pedal pulses but no palpable femoral pulse ipsilaterally. Type I PSA (most common AKA 'complete'), the persistent sciatic artery is main blood supply to the lower limbs (hypoplastic femoral artery), Type II ('incomplete') hypoplasia of the sciatic artery of the thigh and flow dominance by the femoral artery

Crawford's classification of Thoraco-abdominal aneurysms – class I: descending aorta, extending into the abdomen and involving the renal, coeliac and superior mesenteric artery origins, class II: involving most of the descending thoracic and abdominal aorta, class III: involves less than half the descending aorta and part of the abdominal aorta from which the visceral vessels arise, class IV: confined to the abdominal aorta but involving the renal and visceral arteries

Cruveihier's sign – positive cough impulse at saphena varix

DeBakey classification of aortic dissection (also see Stanford Classification) – I: involves ascending and descending aorta (= Stanford A), type II: involves ascending aorta only (= Stanford A), type III: involves descending aorta only, commencing after the origin of the left subclavian artery (= Stanford B)

Delaney-Gonzales AKA Delaney Classification of Popliteal Artery Entrapment Syndrome – Type I normal gastrocnemius displaces artery with looping, Type II, medial head of the gastrocnemius laterally and compresses artery without looping, Type III, accessory slip muscle compression from the medial head of the gastrocnemius, and Type IV, entrapped by the popliteus muscle or by a fibrous band

Dunbar syndrome AKA MALS AKA Median Arcuate Ligament Syndrome AKA Coeliac Artery Compression Syndrome AKA Coeliac axis syndrome AKA Coeliac trunk compression syndrome – Coeliac artery and possibly ganglia pressure due to the median arcuate ligament. Presents with (1) meal pain, (2) weight loss and (3) anterior abdominal bruit

Dunning test – assessment of upper internal carotid artery patency and flow characteristics. Done through the oropharynx at the level of C2 (requires significant patient cooperation)

Eden's Test for **Thoracic Outlet Syndrome (TOS)** AKA Military Brace Test AKA Costoclavicular Test – Supraclavicular compression with shoulder traction (mimicking a military ruck sack/backpack/bergen). Positivity occurs if there is radial pulse compromise during the test.

Ehlers-Danlos syndrome – Genetic connective tissue disorder. May have Arnold–Chiari malformation (structural cerebellar defects), Gorlin sign (tongue to tip of nose), Raynaud's phenomenon, Piezogenic papules (fat-through-dermis papules), Livedo reticularis, 'Cigarette Paper' (atrophic) scars, Peete Syndrome AKA Thoracic Outlet Syndrome, Trendelenburg's sign (hip abductor weakness), Hand signs of Swan neck and Boutonniere deformity of the fingers and Osgood–Schlatter disease AKA apophysitis of the tibial tubercle (inflammed tibial tuberosity patellar ligament). Ehlers-Danlos type IV is associated with aneurysmal disease

Elephant trunk technique – staged cardiovascular procedure where a graft placed at aortic arch/ root repair can be utilised for descending thoraco-abdominal aortic disease further down as a second stage

Fontaine clinical classification of peripheral artery disease – Stage I–Asymptomatic, Stage II–Intermittent claudication [IIa >200m, IIb <200m], Stage III–Rest pain, Stage IV–Ischaemic ulcers or gangrene (which may be dry or humid)

Frank's sign – earlobe crease sign associated with

coronary artery disease and carotid atherosclerosis

Gaiter Ulceration AKA Venous Ulceration – Sign of venous incompetence, sometime associated with Champagne Bottle sign (see above)

Goodman disease AKA abdominal angina

Gruber disease – Cervical rib, (1) just beyond the transverse process, (2) tip between transverse process and first rib, (3) Fibro-cartilaghenous band attached to the first rib (4) Fused to the first rib

Hamming-Vink syndrome AKA Popliteal artery entrapment syndrome – Classified by Love and Whelan and modified by Rich, Types I-VI. Clinical test demonstrated loss of tibial pulse on active plantar flexion or passive dorsiflexion

Hardman index – used in predicting outcomes after open and endovascular repair of ruptured abdominal aortic aneurysms

Harrison and Smyth's syndrome AKA subclavian steal syndrome AKA Contorni syndrome – (1) proximal subclavian artery obstruction, (2) reversed flow in the ipsilateral vertebral artery, and (3) symptoms of cerebral ischaemia

Horner's syndrome – Ptosis, Enophthalmos, Ipsilateral contracted pupil, Ipsilateral anhydrosis

Hutchinson's disease AKA Temporal arteritis AKA Giant cell arteritis – inflammation of large and medium arteries that occurs in >55yr olds, more common in North European women (similar but distinct to Takayasu's arteritis)

Hunter's aneurysm – Popliteal artery aneursym

Kawasaki disease AKA Mucocutaneous lymph node syndrome – Systemic blood vessel inflammation with associated coronary artery aneurysms

Kommerell (Diverticulum) AKA Aberrant subclavian artery AKA aberrant subclavian artery syndrome – aortic arch anomaly

Leriche syndrome AKA Leriche's syndrome AKA aortoiliac occlusive disease – (1) Buttock and thigh claudication, (2) Erectile dysfunction, (3) Absent femoral pulses

Leriche's syndrome Triad – (1) Bilateral lower limb atrophy, (2) Bilateral buttock, hip and thigh pain / claudication, (3) Impotence

Livedoid vasculopathy AKA Livedoid vasculitis AKA Livedo reticularis with summer or winter ulceration AKA Segmental hyalinizing vasculitis AKA PURPLE (acronym) – Chronic venous disease due to venous hypertension or varicosities described as Painful purpuric ulcers with reticular pattern of the lower extremities, Can progress to Atrophie blanche. Sometimes seen in macroglobulinaemia

Lymphoedema praecox AKA Meige's disease AKA Hereditary lymphedema type II – primary lymphoedema in <35yr individuals

Lymphoedema tarda – primary lymphoedema in >35yr individuals

Lymphoedema procedures (below are excisional/ ablative procedures, modern options also include liposuction and lympho-venous anastomotic techniques):

Kondolean Procedure: lymphoedema resection + fascial window

Charles procedure: subcutaneous tissue down to fascia resection

Sistrunk procedure (different to Sistrunk procedure for excision of a thyroglossal cyst): subcutaneous tissue down to fascia resection + skin flaps

Homans-Miller procedure: subcutaneous tissue down to fascia resection + modified cosmetic skin flaps (can be a multi-stage procedure)

Thompson Procedure: considered a Charles-Homan-Miller hybrid, skin flap designed to 'reflect' lymph fluid into the deeper lymph circulation

Marfan syndrome – autosomal dominant connective tissue disorder with increased height, long limbs and digits, scoliosis and increased risk of aneurysms and cardiac valve prolapse. Classified by the Ghent criteria

Martorell's ulcer AKA Ulcus Cruris Hypertonicum – ulcer in lower limbs, typically in females 40-60yr old, associated with systemic hypertension (specifically diastolic)

May-Thurner AKA Cockett's syndrome AKA McMurrich Syndrome AKA nonocclusive iliac vein lesion – Left iliac vein compression from contralateral right common iliac artery (typically against the posterior fifth lumbar vertebral body), a recognised cause of left sided DVTs

Milroy disease AKA early onset lymphoedema type 1A

AKA Nonne-Milroy-Meige syndrome AKA Milroy-Virchow disease AKA and hereditary lymphoedema – hereditary lymphoedema, presents at birth

Meige lymphoedema AKA lymphoedema type 2, AKA Meige disease AKA late-onset lymphoedema – hereditary lymphoedema, presents from the age of 1-35years

Miller vein cuff – support anastomoses between prosthetic conduit and artery

Mönckeberg's arteriosclerosis AKA Mönckeberg's sclerosis AKA Mönckeberg's medial calcific sclerosis or Mönckeberg medial sclerosis – arteriosclerosis and calcification of the tunica media

Nutcracker syndrome – mesoaortic compression, left renal vein compressed by the aorta and SMA

Olivarius carotid sign – Test for internal carotid disease, where a bruit or thrill over one orbit is associated with contralateral internal carotid disease

Parodi Technique – Endovascular stent grafting

Pemberton's sign AKA Superior vena cava syndrome sign– upper mediastinal test mass/blockage test on raising the arms, resulting in (1)facial congestion, (2)cyanosis and (3) respiratory distress (when performed for >1 minute).

Pirogoff angle – angle between the internal jugular and subcalvian vein on both sides

Poiseuille's law of blood – (1) resistance proportional to $1/radius^4$, (2) Flow proportional to $radius^4$ or $1/resistance$. (a) radius, (b) pressure gradient (c) viscosity and (d) vessel length important. Resistance = pressure gradient / flow volume = 8x viscosity (haematocrit) x length/r^4

Peete Syndrome AKA Astley Cooper Disease AKA Adson syndrome AKA Thoracic Outlet Syndrome:

Roos Test for **Thoracic Outlet Syndrome (TOS)** AKA EAST (Elevated Arm Stress Test) – repeatedly open/close fists with arms raised

Saddle embolus – Embolus at the aortic bifurcation

Siegman vein cuff – support anastomoses between heavily calcified small arteries

Stanford classification of aortic dissections (also see DeBakey Classification) – Type A: affects ascending aorta and arch , Type B: begins beyond brachiocephalic vessels distal to the left subclavian artery

Raynaud's syndrome (or primary Raynaud's) – idiopathic hand artery spasm

Saphena varix AKA saphenous varix – Saphenous vein dilatation at its junction with the femoral vein

Scarpa's Triangle AKA Femoral triangle (of Scarpa) – subfascial space bounded by Superior (inguinal ligament), laterally (Sartorius) and medially (adductor longus), medial floor (pectineus, part of the adductor brevis and adductor longus muscles), lateral floor (iliopsoas), roof (fascia lata + cribriform fascia [connective tissue] at the saphenous opening). It contains Femoral nerve, sheath, artery, vein and deep inguinal lymph nodes. Note the saphenous vein penetrates the cribriform facia just above the Allan Burn's ligament AKA Burn's ligament (superior falciform margin of the fascia lata opening)

Takayasu's arteritis AKA Takayasu's disease AKA Aortic arch syndrome AKA Pulseless disease – Large vessel granulomatous vasculitis typically seen in young-to-middle-aged (25-45yr old) Asian women. Initially (1) Inflammatory phase: systemic phase of malaise and illness (2) pulseless phase with peripheral claudication, hypertension, or stenosis to renal of brain arteries. Similar but distinct to Hutchinson's disease AKA Temporal arteritis AKA Giant cell arteritis that occurs in >55yr olds

Trendelenburg Test AKA Brodie-Trendelenburg test – For varicose vein incompetence: Supine patient, leg elevated to drain leg. Tourniquet applied to veins in upper thigh, if on standing the veins all distend then incompetence is at the sapheno-femoral junction, if not, sequentially work down leg (lying down and moving tourniquet down) to assess sites of venous incompetence further down, including above the knee assessing the mid-thigh perforators and below the knee assessing short sapheno-popliteal vein incompetence. Perforators include, Dodd's perforator at the lower 1/3 of the thigh (in Hunter's canal), Boyd's perforator at the knee level (just below the tibial tubercle) and Cockett's perforators at the lower 2/3 of the leg (typically superior, medium and inferior), in addition to medial gastrocnemius perforator and the Fibular perforators (see Perthes' test). Note the venous braches at the sapheno-femoral junction include:(1) Main Saphenous Vein Trunk (perforating the cribriform fascia) and (2) Anterior accessory saphenous AKA Anterolateral, (3) Medial accessory AKA Posteromedial, (4) Superficial external pudendal, (5) Superficial circumflex iliac, (6) Superficial inferior epigastric (7) Deep external pudendal. i.e 2 external pudendals, 2 accessories, circumflex iliac and epigastric

Taylor patch – between prosthetic conduit and artery. Consists of a longer arteriotomy with a U-shaped slit on the graft to produce minimal angulation

St Mary's Hybrid Thoraco-abdominbal Aneurysm (TAAA) repair – Hybrid open-endovascular technique (combined or staged), first bypassing visceral aortic side branches so that their origins can be covered with a stent-graft thereby achieving total aneurysm exclusion. (The technique was primarily designed for early stent-grafts that could not accommodate visceral aortic branches)

St Mary's vein Boot AKA Tyrell-Wolfe Boot – Hybrid between Miller cuff and Taylor patch, vein patch with U-shaped slit and longer arteriotomy to join prosthetic conduit to artery

Perthes' test – distal calf, venous incompetent perforator test, similar set-up to the Trendelenburg Test AKA Brodie-Trendelenburg test. However once tourniquet is applied to the upper thigh, patient is stood up and tourniquet gently released, and patient asked to repeatedly 'tip-toe'. If the lower calf perforators are patent and the calf muscles are functioning well, then the prominent lower calf veins become less 'pressured'

Phlegmasia cerulea dolens AKA Blue Ileofemoral DVT syndrome – Blue, painful, oedematous

Phlegmasia alba dolens AKA milk white leg AKA White **Ileofemoral DVT syndrome** – white, painful, oedematous

VASS (Vascular access steal syndrome) AKA DASS (dialysis-associated steal syndrome) – preferential fistula flow when compared to native vessel. Can present with blue, cold, painful limb (occasionally with ulceration)

Virchow's triad – factors associated with thrombosis: (1)

Vessel wall (endothelial function/ dysfunction/ injury), (2) Flow (haemodynamic stasis/ turbulence), (3) Clotting (systemic status/ hypercoagulability)

White toe syndrome – Raynaud's phenomenon in the foot

Wegener's granulomatosis AKA Granulomatosis with polyangiitis – Systemic autoimmune vasculitis affecting small and medium-sized vessels (typically in the lungs and kidneys), has a known association with Pyoderma gangrenosum

Wright's Test for **Thoracic Outlet Syndrome (TOS)** AKA Hyperabduction Test – Hyperadduct shoulder when shoulder and elbow both resting at 90^0. Positivity occurs if there is radial pulse compromise during the test.

ABOUT THE AUTHOR

Hutan Ashrafian, Bsc Hons, MBBS, MRCS, MBA, PhD is a scientist, surgeon, philosopher and historian.

He is currently lecturer in surgery at Imperial College London and senior surgeon registrar at Chelsea and Westminster Hospital in London. Awarded the Arris and Gale Lectureship by the Royal College of Surgeons of England and the Hunterian Prize, he leads a team focusing on the development of innovative technological, digital, pharmaceutical and economic strategies to resolve the global healthcare burden of obesity, metabolic syndrome and cancer.

His clinical experience includes senior houseman at the Royal Brompton, Royal National Orthopaedic, Royal London Emergency Department and St Mary's (Imperial Healthcare NHS Trust) Hospitals. He subsequently completed registrarships in paediatric cardiothoracic surgery at Great Ormond Street Hospital and metabolic medicine, adult cardiothoracic and general surgery at Imperial Healthcare NHS Trust. He concluded his general surgical registrar training at Chelsea and Westminster Hospital in upper gastrointestinal and Bariatric-Metabolic surgery.